Client Profiles in Nursing

Child Health

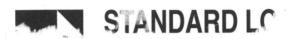 STANDARD L

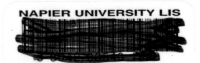

Client Profiles in Nursing

Child Health

Edited by

Gill Campbell BEd(Hons) DPSN RGN RSCN

School of Health and Social Care
University of Portsmouth

Ruth Sadik RSCN RGN BA(Hons) MSc RNT RCNT CertEd

School of Health Studies
University of Portsmouth

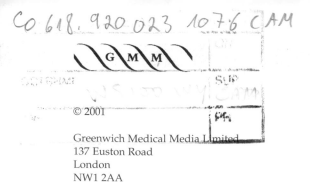

© 2001

Greenwich Medical Media Limited
137 Euston Road
London
NW1 2AA

ISBN 1 84110 013 7

First published 2001

Visit our website at:
www.greenwich-medical.co.uk

Distributed worldwide by Plymbridge Distributors Ltd

Typeset by Phoenix Photosetting, Chatham, Kent
Printed by Ashford Colour Press Ltd, Hants

Contents

Contents

This series of learning aids has been designed for use by pre-registration student nurses, their assessors, nurse educationalists and healthcare support workers undertaking NVQ Level 3. The aim of the series is to simulate as far as possible in writing the kinds of complex human situations that registered and unregistered practitioners are likely to encounter in the course of their work and which will influence assessment and decision-making in terms of nursing management.

Each volume may be used for revision purposes, to generate ideas about producing case profiles or as a basis for compiling questions for use with learners.

The authors are all highly experienced registered nurses, who have compiled the profiles utilising their areas of specialist knowledge and professional experience. Truth, as the saying goes, is stranger than fiction, and it is hoped that the cases reflect this perversity, which most clinical nurses will recognise at once to be the case!

Volume 2 has been written with the nursing of children and infants in mind and there has been a deliberate attempt to present a balanced range of ages, ethnic backgrounds, gender, social circumstances, acute and chronic conditions, and healthcare settings (community and hospital) to stimulate readers' thinking and to focus thought away from purely pathological matters. The Editors have attempted to reflect the reality of the National Health Service, in which the majority of nursing occurs with chronic conditions and in primary care or community settings. Health promotion is also emphasised, reflecting contemporary health policy.

The questions posed range from those that are short and descriptive based on anatomy and physiology, to very complex management questions. The latter will require some time to identify the main issues and subsequently to prioritise these.

Each case profile consists of a scenario, questions and model answers, a reference list and suggestions for further reading.

Tinuade Okubadejo
MSc BSc (Hons) PGCEA RN RM PGDip HV
Southampton Community NHS Trust
Southampton

How to use this book for revision

It is suggested that readers will need to have the following to hand: a nursing or medical dictionary, a pharmacology textbook, and an anatomy and physiology textbook to maximise their use of time.

The index outlines the main topic areas for each case profile. It is assumed that the reader who wishes to use this volume for revision purposes will have learned the relevant topic area before answering the questions!

Each scenario should be read through carefully, with notes made of the main points. The questions should then be read. The clockface logo by each question gives an estimate of the time-scale involved for thinking about and planning the answer. Whenever you are ready, turn over the page to view the answers. You may wish to develop answers by further reading. Questions can also be dealt with one at a time or in a block.

Further volumes will deal with more paediatric nursing and care of the adult patient. If you would like to submit profiles for inclusion in future volumes in this series, the Editors would be delighted to hear from you.

The Editors and authors very much hope that readers will enjoy working with this book since they believe that learning is much easier when the mind is having fun! Happy learning!

Tinuade Okubadejo
May 2001

Abbreviations and symbols

ABC	Airway, breathing and circulation
BP	blood pressure
CRT	Capillary refill time
FBC	Full blood count
GP	general practitioner
IV	intravenous
NBM	Nil by mouth
SaO$_2$	Partial saturation of arterial oxygen
U/E	Urea and electrolytes

Debbi Atkinson BSc(Hons), RGN, RN(Child), DipHE, FAETC
Senior Staff Nurse
Intensive Care Unit
Queen Alexandra Hospital
Portsmouth, UK

Leigh F Caws MSc, RGN, RSCN, DipN(Lond), CertED(F.E)
Senior Lecturer in Child Health
University of Portsmouth, UK

Dawn Cowley Dip, H.E. Registered Nurse/Child
Staff Nurse
Children's Unit
St Mary Hospital
Portsmouth
Hants, UK

Gill Campbell, RN, RSCN, DPSN, BEd(Hons)
Senior Lecturer in Child Health and Child Protection
School of Health and Social Care
University of Portsmouth
St George's Building
Portsmouth, UK

Lucy Davies Dip, HE/RN(mental health)
Community Psychiatric Nurse
Southsea
Hants, UK

Caroline Elliot, BSc(Hons), RSCN, SRN
Paediatric Resuscitation Officer
Southampton University Hospitals Trust
Southampton, UK

Tessa Horlock
Staff Nurse
St Marys Hospital
Portsmouth, UK

Angela Jones RSCN
Community Childrens Nurse
Cosham Health Centre
Portsmouth, UK

Client profiles in nursing: child health

Wendy H Jones, BN, DANS, PGDip(ED), RGN, RSCN, OND
Senior Lecturer
University of Portsmouth
Old Portsmouth, UK

Jane McConochie, BSc(Hons), Nursing Studies, ENB Higher Award, City &
Guilds 730, SRN, RSCN
Senior Staff Nurse
G1 Ward
Queen Alexandra Hospital
Cosham, UK

Ruth Sadik RSCN, RN, BA(Hons), MSc(Child Health), RNT, RCNT
Child Branch Co-ordinator
School of Health Studies
Portsmouth University
Queen Alexandra Hospital
Portsmouth, UK

Sarah D Standley, Dip.H.E Registered Nurse/Child
'D' Grade Staff Nurse
Childrens Unit
St Mary's Hospital
Portsmouth, UK

Christine Ward SRN, RSCN, ENB 148
Senior Sister Paediatric Neurosurgery
Wessex Neuro Centre
Southampton University Hospital NHS Trust
Southampton, UK

Joy Ward RSCN
Children's Community Nurse
Brazmar Avenue
East Cosham
Portsmouth, UK

Cyanotic heart lesion: resuscitation

Caroline Elliott

Rahul is the second child of Meeta and Ali Kahn. His brother Zain is now 2 years old and Meeta required treatment for postnatal depression after Zain's birth. She does not speak English but can understand a limited amount.

Rahul was born at home following a normal full-term delivery and weighed 3.5 kg. Meeta commenced breastfeeding her newborn but, 36 h later, the midwife, Katy, when making her postnatal visit, was concerned that Rahul was not feeding well and was grunting, which Meeta told her started the previous night. Following discussion with the GP trainee over the phone, admission was arranged to the emergency admissions ward for assessment.

Meeta, tearful and cradling Rahul to her bosom, walked with a straddling gait (following her episiotomy) onto the ward. Katy accompanied her, and Ali, who speaks English, is on his way.

On examination, Rahul has:

- Slate grey colour
- Shallow irregular slow respirations
- Unobtainable oxygen saturation level
- Capillary refill > 12 s
- Heart rate of 125 beats min^{-1} and temperature of 37.2°C
- He is currently anuric
- He is unconscious and hypotonic

Following investigation Rahul has:

- Blood glucose < 0.5 mmol l^{-1} (see Profile 12, Gareth Jones)
- Arterial blood pH 6.8 (normal 7.29–7.45) (Campbell & Glasper, 1995)

Preliminary cardiac ultrasound reveals severe co-arctation of the aorta and hypoplastic left ventricle.

Rahul is oxygenated, bagged and intubated. IV and intra-osseous access are gained for administration of resuscitation drugs, vasodilators, inotropes and fluids. Monitoring includes cardiac, non-invasive BP and the partial saturation of arterial oxygen (SaO$_2$). The portable incubator/ventilator is prepared before transfer of Rahul to the regional cardiac centre in a nearby city. Ali has now arrived and following an explanation of Rahul's condition, he and his wife follow the ambulance by car.

Question one: Briefly describe the fetal circulation and the changes that take place following birth.

15 minutes

Question two: With reference to Rahul, describe his cardiac abnormality.

15 minutes

Question three: What preparations would one undertake for the expected admission of Rahul, giving a brief rationale?

30 minutes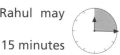

Question four: Precalculate the resuscitation drugs/fluids Rahul may require.

15 minutes

Time Allowance: **1 hour 15 minutes**

Answer to question one:
Briefly describe the fetal circulation and the changes that take place following birth.

Fetal blood, oxygenated in the placenta, enters the fetus through the umbilical vein. Blood enters the ductus venosus, bypasses the hepatic circulation and flows into the inferior vena cava. Once in the right atrium, it is diverted toward the atrial septum and flows through the foramen ovale into the left atria. Blood then passes through the left ventricle and ascending aorta to perfuse the head and upper extremities. This pathway allows the best-oxygenated blood from the placenta to perfuse the fetal brain. Venous blood from the head and upper extremities returns to the fetal heart through the superior vena cava, enters the right atrium and right ventricle, and flows into the pulmonary artery. Since pulmonary vascular resistance is high, the blood is diverted through the ductus arteriosus into the descending aorta. Ultimately much of this blood returns to the placenta through the umbilical arteries (Wong et al., 1999). This is clearly seen in Figure 1.1.

Once the infant is born, the lungs expand and the infant is responsible for his own oxygenation. The ductus arteriosus and foramen ovale are no longer required.

A rise in the neonatal arterial oxygen tension is thought to be the most important stimulus to ductal constriction and functional closure is usually produced within 10–24 h following a full-term birth (Hazinski, 1999).

The fall in pulmonary vascular resistance produces a corresponding fall in right ventricular and atrial pressures and, therefore, the foramen ovale closes as left atrial pressure exceeds right atrial pressure (Hazinski, 1999).

Client profiles in nursing: child health

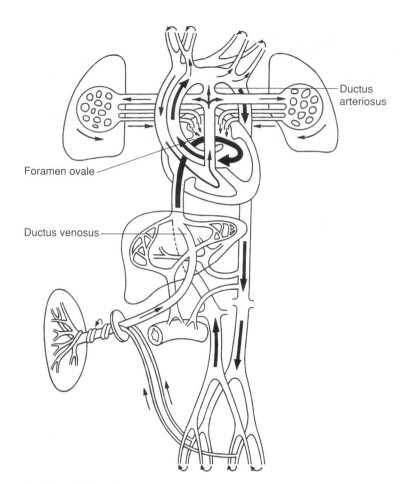

Ductus
arteriosus

Foramen ovale

Ductus venosus

Figure 1.1. Fetal circulation.

Answer to question two:
With reference to Rahul, briefly describe his cardiac abnormality.

Rahul has two congenital cardiac abnormalities:

- Hypoplastic left ventricle: according to Suddaby & Grenier (1999), this has an incidence rate of 2%. It refers to the underdevelopment of the left side of the heart. The aorta also is minute and blood can only reach the rest of the body through the ductus arteriosus. Initially, this causes mild cyanosis but as the ductus arteriosus closes, there is progressive deterioration with increasing cyanosis and decreasing cardiac output, leading to cardiovascular collapse (Figure 1.2)
- Co-arctation of the aorta: this condition has an incidence rate of 12% (Suddaby & Grenier, 1999). It involves localized narrowing of the aorta close to the insertion of the ductus arteriosus. The left ventricle has to pump at a higher pressure to force the blood through the narrowed area. However, this is impossible with an hypoplastic left ventricle. Severe co-arctation in itself causes the baby to be breathless, unable to feed normally and to become shocked (Figure 1.3)

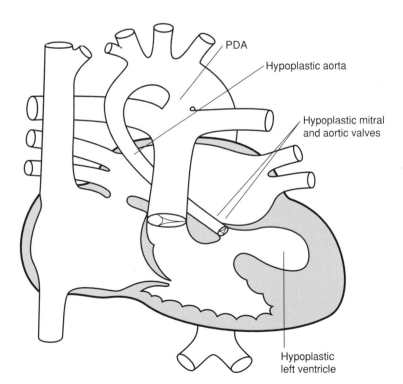

Figure 1.2. Hypoplastic left ventricle.

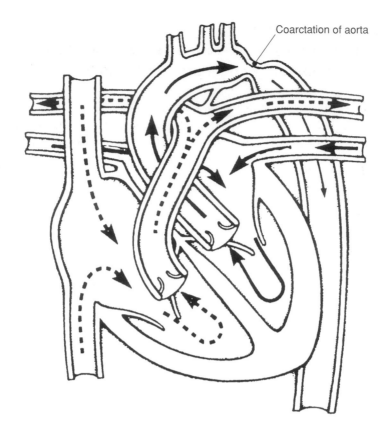

Coarctation of aorta

Figure 1.3. Co-arctation of the aorta.

Answer to question three:
What preparations would one undertake for the expected admission of Rahul, giving a brief rationale?

In readiness for the arrival of Rahul, the nurse would prepare a resuscitaire with heat and light to provide a controlled environment and temperature.

The remaining equipment is assembled following an airway, breathing and circulation (ABC) protocol based on a hierarchy of need (Advanced Life Support Group, 1997).

Airway and breathing:

- Oxygen and infant mask with reservoir
- Resuscitation bag (500 ml) and mask (0,0/1) with reservoir
- Ayres' T-piece with peak inspiratory pressure set to 20 cm
- Suction – set at a maximum of 10 kPa with 6-Fg catheters and a mini-yankaue sucker for removal of secretions or debris from Rahul's airway
- Straight short bladed (0,1) laryngoscope
- Introducer and stethoscope
- Endotracheal tubes – 2.5, 3.0 and 3.5 mm
- Paediatric Magill's forceps to introduce the tube
- Suture (3/0), elastoplast, waterproof adhesive tape, tincture of benzoin compound for skin preparation
- 6-Fg nasogastric tube, tape and bag for drainage
- Pulse oximeter with sensor suitable for < 10 kg

Circulation:

- Cardiorator, non-invasive BP monitor
- IV and intra-osseous access – fluids/drugs
- Arterial catheter of appropriate size
- Blood glucose meter
- Blood sample bottles for full blood count, urea and electrolytes, C-reactive protein and cultures

Answer to question four:
Precalculate the resuscitation drugs/fluids Rahul may require.

Table 1.1 shows examples of the fluid and drugs that Rahul may be prescribed by the medical staff.

Table 1.1. Possible fluid and drugs prescribed by medical staff.

Drug/fluid	Reason	Dose (ml kg⁻¹)	Prescribed dose for Rahul (ml)
Normal saline (0.9%)	correct hypovolaemia	20	70
Glucose	correct hypoglycaemia	5	17.5
Sodium bicarbonate (4.2%)	correct acidosis	1 mmol	7
Prostin infusion	maintain patency of ductus arteriosus	0.05 mcg⁻¹ kg min⁻¹	0.175 mcg min⁻¹
Dobutamine	increase the contraction of the heart muscle	2.5 mcg⁻¹ kg min⁻¹	8.75 mcg min⁻¹
Adrenaline:	increases heart rate and contractility:		
First dose	1:10 000	0.1	0.35
Second dose	1:1000	0.1	0.35

NB: Bicarbonate when administered with calcium will cause a precipitation, so care should be taken that these two solutions are administered separately. Bicarbonate will also inactivate dopamine and adrenaline so the same precaution must apply.

(Hazinski, 1999)

References

Advanced Life Support Group (1997). *Advanced Paediatric Life Support*, 2nd edn. London: BMJ Publ.

Campbell, S., & Glasper, E. A. (eds) (1995). *Whaley and Wong's Children's Nursing*. London: Mosby.

Hazinski, M. F. (1999). *Manual of Pediatric Critical Care*. London: Mosby.

Suddaby, E. C., & Grenier, M. A. (1999). The embryology of congenital heart defects. *Pediatric Nursing*, 25, 499–505.

Wong, D., Hockenberry-Eaton, M., Wilson, D., Winkelstein, M. L., Ahmann, E., & DiVito-Thomas, P. (1999). *Whaley and Wong's Nursing Care of Infants and Children*, 6th edn. St Louis: Mosby.

Further reading

Pediheart Website (2000, accessed 31 July 2000). Practitioners' site [http://www.pediheart.org/practitioners/index.htm].

Infant with tracheo-oesophageal fistula

Gill Campbell and Ruth Sadik

Michael Connolly was born at full-term to Denise and James. He is their second child, Michael having an older sister, Katy, who is 4 years old. At birth he was noticed to be very 'bubbly' and required oral and naso-pharyngeal suction. Michael was put to the breast soon after birth but this had to be abandoned as he quickly started coughing and spluttering. An attempt to pass a nasogastric tube was unsuccessful and Michael was subsequently diagnosed as having a tracheo-oesophageal fistula and oesophageal atresia. Denise and James were initially devastated by the news having had no previous inclination that they were not expecting a normal healthy baby. It was explained to them that in Michael's case the upper oesophagus ended in a blind pouch while the lower oesophagus was connected to the trachea. Michael required surgery to allow him to feed and to prevent gastric contents spilling out into the trachea and lungs. An IV infusion was commenced to correct Michael's electrolyte imbalance and to provide hydration. An oesophagostomy and percutaneous endo-scopic gastrostomy (PEG) with a skin-level device (button) were performed on the second day of life. James and Denise were told that this was only the first operation that Michael would require and that the stoma on Michael's neck was to drain any saliva and food from his mouth while the stoma in his abdominal wall led directly to his stomach and was used for feeding Michael. It was explained to Denise that she would need to feed Michael orally and via the gastrostomy simultaneously.

Question one: Explain the common types of tracheo-oesophageal fistulae in infancy.

20 minutes

Question two: Outline the care that Michael will require pre-operatively.

30 minutes

Question three: Discuss the rationale for feeding Michael orally and via the gastrostomy simultaneously.

10 minutes

Question four: Explain the information that Michael's family will need to care for him at home.

15 minutes

Time Allowance: **1 hour 15 minutes**

Answer to question one:
Explain the common types of tracheo-oesophageal fistulae in infancy.

Tracheo-oesophageal atresia with or without a fistula is a congenital abnormality of the trachea (TOA/TOF) (Figure 2.1). It affects ~1:3000 births. In 50% of cases (Spitz, 1993), it is associated with VATER syndrome, a chromosomal abnormality resulting in a group of conditions occurring together:

V vertebral defects
A anal atresia
T tracheo-oesophageal fistula
E (o)esophageal atresia
R renal or radial dysplasia

Of the above types, the most common presentation is atresia of the oesophagus with an associated distal tracheo-oesophageal fistula (c), most of which could not be totally repaired at initial surgery (Spitz *et al.*, 1993).

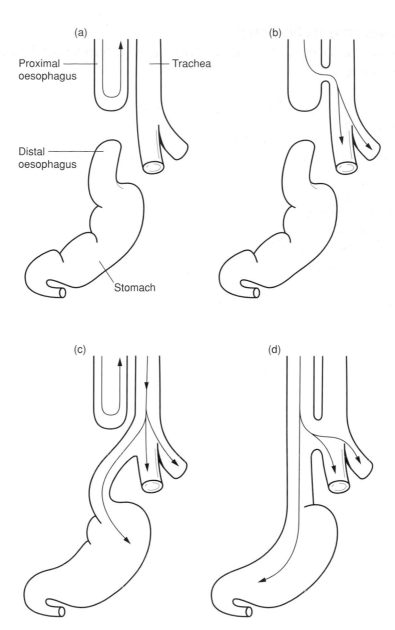

Figure 2.1. Types of tracheo-oesophageal abnormality.

Answer to question two:
Outline the care that Michael will require pre-operatively.

Although Michael required surgery soon after birth, it was more important that he was physiologically stable (Spitz *et al.*, 1993). In other cases, there may be longer time before surgery. The main aim of preoperative care is to protect the airway and prevent aspiration pneumonia. This is achieved in Michael's case by him being nursed head-up. A fine-bored, radio-opaque Replogle tube was passed into the upper pouch, which will remain on constant low-pressure suction (known as a sump drain) (Ein *et al.*, 1993). The tube will require regular flushing to ensure patency. To maintain Michael's body temperature and secretion liquidity, he may be nursed in a warm, humid environment, probably via an incubator. The loosening of secretions may lead to Michael requiring nasal and oral suction. He will also require chest physiotherapy and antibiotics to prevent further complications.

Michael was physiologically relatively stable and required an IV infusion merely to provide hydration pre-theatre. In other cases, several days of enteral feeding may be required. The nurse's role will be to monitor the infusion and the cannula site for signs of extravasation or infection.

Family-centred care dictates parental involvement in all aspects of Michael's care giving and decision-making (Casey, 1997). The children's nurse will, there-fore, provide the opportunity for James and Denise to share their thoughts, fears and anxieties as regards their son's condition and progress with appropri-ate healthcare professionals. Campbell and Glasper (1995) suggested that this support involves understanding the parents need to comprehend their situa-tion.

Some infants born with TOF require transferring to regional centres for surgery, where the expertise in these cases is consolidated. If this is the case with Michael, Denise and James will need to be informed and prepared. Chaplen (1997) emphasized the need to inform the parents about oesophagos-tomies and gastrostomies pre-operatively. This would also include a rationale for sham feeding.

Answer to question three:
Discuss the rationale for feeding Michael orally and via the gastrostomy simultaneously.

The process of feeding Michael simultaneously via his mouth and gastrostomy is known as 'sham' feeding. During this procedure, the feed given orally will be collected via the oesophagostomy into a receptacle. It, therefore, plays no nutritional role in feeding. However, it does acquaint Michael with the taste and sensation of food in his mouth and the processes of sucking and swallowing. The feed given via gastrostomy will also establish the link between Michael's sucking and swallowing and the sensation of gastric filling. Campbell and Glasper (1995) suggested that it might be difficult to establish oral feeding post-total correction if sham feeding has not occurred as the links between sucking and swallowing and gastric filling will not have been established. Michael also needs to retain the sensation of sucking as this has a non-nutritive stress-relieving function (Medoff-Cooper et al., 1989).

Answer to question four:
Explain the information that Michael's family will need to care for him at home.

The need for parental information and involvement has been understood for many years, but has more recently been highlighted by the Department of Health, which states: 'You and your child have the right to be given an explanation of any treatment proposed, including the benefits, risks and alternatives, before you decide whether you will agree to it' (1996: 13). Denise and James will be told it is likely to be 6–12 months before Michael's final operation (Spitz *et al.*, 1993).

Michael will need to continue his chest physiotherapy at home and his parents may need to be taught how to perform this themselves. It is customary for the community physiotherapist to be involved with the family throughout (Cluroe, 1989). Antibiotics will also be continued to prevent infections.

Both parents should demonstrate their competence at sham feeding before Michael is discharged and will need advice about both of the stomas. The skin around both stomas is prone to soreness, which can be lessened by the application of a thin layer of petroleum jelly. There is also the possibility of over granulation of the stoma site and meticulous skin care, including cleaning the skin site and rotating the device daily, have been identified by Chaplen (1997) as being important facts for parental information.

Nutritionally Michael will require the same diet as any other infant of his age. This will include weaning at the appropriate time of 4 months. The parents will need to be confident in attaching the feeding apparatus to the button. If the tube should block, Denise and James should be instructed to irrigate the tube with 1 ml normal saline (Campbell & Glasper, 1995). If the device is inadvertently removed, the parents should be instructed not to panic but to insert the spare and to report to the nearest hospital. Turner and Watson (1990) identified these issues as being of major concern to the parents.

The community nursing team or GP would generally supply the supplies required for the gastrostomy.

References

Campbell, S., & Glasper, E. A. (eds) (1995). *Whaley and Wong's Children's Nursing*. London: Mosby.

Chaplen, C. (1997). Parents views of caring for children with gastrostomies. *British Journal of Nursing*, 6, 34–38.

Cluroe, S. (1989). Congenital oesophageal abnormalities. *Nursing*, 3, 20–23.

Department of Health (1996). *NHS The Patient's Charter: Services for Children and Young People*. London: HMSO.

Medoff-Cooper, B., Weininger, S., & Zukowsky, K. (1989). Neonatal sucking as a clinical assessment tool: preliminary findings. *Nursing Research*, 38, 162–164.

Spitz, L. (1993). Eosophageal atresia and tracheoesophageal fistula in children. *Current Opinions in Pediatrics*, 5, 347–352.

Spitz, L., Kiely, E., Brereton, R., & Drake, D. (1993). Management of esophageal atresia. *World Journal of Surgery*, 17, 296–300.

Useful information

http://www.aafp.org/afp/990215ap/910.html
http://www.tofs.ndirect.co.uk
TOF Society, St George's Centre, 91 Victoria Road, Netherfield, Nottingham NG4 2NN, UK.

Tracheo-oesophageal fistula

Hydrocephalus

Christine Ward

Mandy and Brian Silvers had two children, a 4-year-old son called Sam and a 2-year-old daughter named Hannah. The whole family were delighted when they found out that they were to have a new addition. Jane was born 2 months ago. It was an easy birth for Mandy, and Brian was thrilled to have another daughter. Jane stayed in hospital for 24 h after the routine assessment had been made on Jane, in which all was normal. Mandy decided to bottle-feed Jane.

For the first week of life Jane was the perfect baby and Sam and Hannah made a lot of fuss of her. However, over the next couple of days Jane became restless and irritable. Mandy was not too concerned as she had just moved Jane into her own room and was sure that it was just the new surroundings. Mandy initially decided to persevere with Jane being in her own room; however, she also noticed that Jane was not taking her feeds very well. She seemed to be uninterested in her bottles, cried when she was picked up and appeared unable to settle.

A week passed and Jane had not really improved. The whole family was becoming distressed as Jane was waking in the night and not settling again. Mandy made an appointment with the Health Visitor, Maureen, for the next day.

When Maureen arrived, Jane, who by now was 3 weeks old, was crying a high-pitched cry and Mandy was almost at the end of her tether. Maureen noticed that Jane had 'sunset eyes' (Figure 3.1).

When Maureen measured Jane's head circumference, she was concerned that the measurement was 40 cm, which is > 97th centile, while length and weight were both just below the 50th.

Maureen arranged an appointment with the GP, who subsequently arranged for Jane to be admitted to hospital for investigations into hydrocephalus.

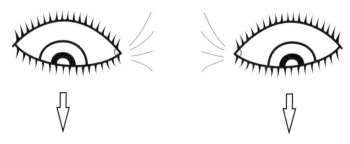

Figure 3.1. 'Sunset eyes'.

Question one: What is hydrocephalus?

15 minutes

Question two: Describe the flow of cerebrospinal fluid.

15 minutes

Question three: Describe the possible causes of Jane's hydrocephalus.

15 minutes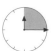

Question four: What information would one need to know to explain to the parents the signs and symptoms that Jane is displaying?

15 minutes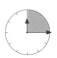

Time Allowance: **1 hour**

Answer to question one:
What is hydrocephalus?

The term 'hydrocephalus' comes from two Greek words meaning water on the head. The watery fluid is called cerebrospinal fluid (CSF). Hydrocephalus is caused by an imbalance between the production and absorption of CSF within the ventricular system due to an obstruction of CSF circulation. This results in an accumulation of fluid. As the sutures of the infant's cranium are still patent, the fluid accumulation splays them, resulting in an enlarged cranium (Donaghy, 1993).

Answer to question two:
Describe the flow of cerebrospinal fluid.

The choroid plexus within the four communicating ventricles of the brain produces the CSF. The choroid plexus is a highly vascular structure lining the floor of the lateral ventricle and roof of the third and fourth ventricles up to the subarachnoid space, which surrounds the brain and spinal cord.

The CSF provides a protective cushion for the brain and helps regulate the intracranial pressure (ICP). It also provides nutrients needed for the physiological functioning and a mechanism for removing waste products from the central nervous system.

The CSF flows from the lateral ventricles into the third ventricle through the foramen of Munro. It then passes from the third to the fourth ventricle via the aqueduct of Sylvius. The fluid leaves the fourth ventricle and enters the subarachnoid space via the foramen of Luschka and then the foramen of Magendie. The CSF leaving the foramen of Magendie circulates into the cisterna and down the spinal cord (Kapit & Elson, 1998) (Figure 3.2).

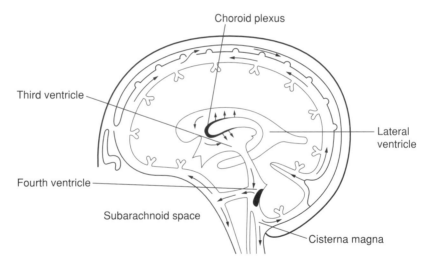

Figure 3.2. CSF flow.

Answer to question three:
Describe the possible causes of Jane's hydrocephalus.

Hydrocephalus can be either communicating or non-communicating. Communicating hydrocephalus is caused by an obstruction of CSF at the sub-arachnoid cisterna, therefore obstructing the flow of CSF through the ventricular pathways. A range of conditions, such as inflammation, congenital abnormalities, tumours or absorption problems, can cause this (Detwiler *et al.*, 1999). The obstruction causes a fluid build up, which leads to distension of the ventricles.

Non-communicating hydrocephalus is caused by an obstruction in the ventricular system, such as aqueduct stenosis, impaired development of the ventricles and obstruction at the foramen of Munro and outlets of the fourth ventricle (Wong *et al.*, 1999).

Answer to question four:
What information would one need to know to explain to the parents the signs and symptoms that Jane is displaying?

The signs and symptoms of raised ICP can be explained through the Munroe–Kellie hypothesis, which states that the sum of all the volume compartments within the skull is constant. The skull compartment volumes are:

- Brain and glial tissue: 70%
- CSF: 10%
- Blood: 10%
- Interstitial fluid: 10%

If the volume of one compartment changes, then the other volumes must compensate. The normal CSF pressures are (University of Adelaide, 2000):

- Infant: 40–50 mmH$_2$O
- Child: 40–100 mmH$_2$O

The first of these to compensate is CSF. As the pressure increases, the CSF moves from the intracranial vault to the dural sac. Eventually, this ceases and the ventricles collapse. If the ICP rises above the maximum limit of 50 mmH$_2$O (for Jane), a shift in brain structure or an interruption to blood flow occurs. Interruption to blood flow causes a second major problem. As ICP rises, cerebral blood flow continues, albeit inefficiently. When ICP equals the systemic arterial pressure, blood flow ceases completely and neural death ensues (Hazinski, 1999).

Jane has a developmental defect that causes the flow of CSF in the brain to become obstructed. This leads to the ventricles in the brain enlarging and swelling. As Jane's cranium is still very soft and the sutures have not yet fused, her skull has expanded and, as a result, the fontanelles become tense and bulging. The increased ICP distorts the cranium, stretching the skin over the forehead giving the appearance of 'sunset eyes' (Figure 3.1). Wong et al. (1999) attributed this to pressure on the techtum of the mesencephalon from the third ventricle or the orbital roof.

As the pressure within the skull increases, the bones thin and separate at the sutures. If the skull is lightly tapped, the sound made is reminiscent of a 'cracked pot', also known as MacEwen's sign (Detwiler et al., 1999).

Rising ICP causes disruption of brain stem functions that causes Jane to become irritable with a typical high-pitched cry, lethargic and uninterested in her feeds.

Treatment for Jane's condition is to insert an intracranial shunt between the ventricles and either the peritoneum or right ventricle to allow the accumulated fluid to drain (Wong et al., 1999). If surgery is performed before brain function has been compromised, then Jane's prognosis is excellent, with a good chance that she will lead a happy, normal life (Detwiler et al., 1999).

References

Detwiler, P. W., Porter, R. W., & Rekate, H. C. (1999). Hydrocephalus – clinical features and management. In M. D. Choux, C. Rocco, A. D. Hockley, & M. L. Walker (eds), *Pediatric Neurosurgery* (253–271). New York: Churchill Livingstone.

Donaghy, L. S. (1993). Hydrocephalus. *Canadian Journal of Medical Radiation Technology, 24,* 13–17.

Hazinski, M. F. (1999). *Manual of Pediatric Critical Care.* London: Mosby.

Kapit, W., & Elson, L. (1998). *The Anatomy Coloring Book,* 2nd edn. London: Addison-Wesley.

Wong, D. L., Hockenberry-Eaton, M., Wilson, D., Winkelstein, M. L., Ahmann, E., & DiVito-Thomas, P. A. (1999). *Whaley and Wong's Nursing Care of Infants and Children,* 6th edn. St Louis: Mosby.

University of Adelaide (n.d., accessed 29 March 2000). Hydrocephalus [http://www.health.adelaide.edu.au/paed-neuro/hydro.html].

Further reading

May, L., & Carter, B. (1995). *Child Health Care Nursing: Concepts, Theories and Practice.* Oxford: Blackwells.

Rekate, H. L. (1997). Recent advances in understanding and treatment of hydrocephalus. *Seminars in Pediatric Neurology, 4,* 167–178.

Shiminski, M. T., & Disabato, J. (1994). Current trends in the diagnosis and management of hydrocephalus in children. *Journal of Pediatric Nursing: Nursing Care of Children and Families, 9,* 74–82.

Acute bronchiolitis

Gill Campbell

Michael Smith is the second son of Louise and Barry Smith, their elder son, James being 2 years old. Michael was born at full-term and is now 3 months old. He was well until 3 days ago when he presented with a cough, snuffles and a difficulty in breathing. Louise took Michael to the GP who diagnosed him as suffering from acute bronchiolitis. He organized admission to the childrens' ward of the local hospital. On admission, Michael was pale and tachypnoeic (respiration rate = 60 breaths min^{-1}) and his respirations were shallow. He was mildly pyrexial with a temperature of 38°C. He had an audible wheeze and appeared mildly dehydrated. Both parents, who appeared anxious and concerned, accompanied Michael. James was also with them and he appeared quiet and miserable with an obvious cold. Michael was admitted to the ward and Louise explained that he had not been feeding well for the past 24 h, saying, 'he just can't suck with this runny nose'. Michael weighed 5.0 kg, which was on the 10th centile, and his length was 59 cm, which was above the 10th centile. He had marked retractions and appeared uninterested. An IV infusion was commenced as Michael was mildly dehydrated and not taking sufficient fluids orally. He was commenced on humidified oxygen therapy at 7 l min^{-1} via a headbox and a pulse oximeter was attached to his great toe to monitor oxygen saturation levels.

Question one: Outline the underlying pathophysiology of bronchiolitis.
10 minutes

Question two: Discuss the nursing care that Michael will need during his hospital stay.
25 minutes

Time Allocation: **35 minutes**

Client profiles in nursing: child health

Answer to question one:
Outline the underlying pathophysiology of bronchiolitis.

Bronchiolitis is a disease found in infants and children < 2 years of age. It is caused by inflammation of the small bronchioles. A virus, the most common one being respiratory syncytial virus (RSV), usually causes the inflammation. The virus attaches itself to the epithelial cells in the respiratory tract. Oedema and necrosis can occur as part of the inflammatory response. This, in turn, can cause collapse of the alveoli or, if the obstruction is incomplete, for hyper-inflation as air is trapped beyond the obstruction (Campbell & Glasper, 1995; Gould, 1997).

At birth, the respiratory system is immature and it is only as the baby grows that the bronchioles increase in size and the alveoli increase in number (Moules & Ramsay, 1998). This increases the risk of blockage of the small airways and alveoli by secretions or oedema. A baby can only breath through the nose for the first 4 weeks of life. If the nasal passages become blocked by secretions, the baby will become apnoeic (Moules & Ramsay, 1998).

Answer to question two:
Discuss the nursing care that Michael will need during his hospital stay.

The treatment for Michael is predominantly supportive. The nurse should ensure that Michael is nursed in a cubicle on his own to reduce the risk of cross-infection by direct contact. Hand washing and using gloves when coming into contact with Michael's secretions should eliminate the risk to others.

Michael is receiving humidified oxygen. It is important for the nurse to check the humidifier regularly as dry oxygen, if delivered, would increase the viscosity of the secretions and would exacerbate Michael's problems. The effect of the oxygen should be monitored by assessing Michael's pulse, respiratory rate and pattern and it should be ensured that Michael's skin does not become grey or mottled (Sadik & Elliott, 1999). The oxygen should not be pointed directly at Michael as this may cause blood to move from the peripheral circulation to the central circulation with subsequent bradycardia (Campbell & Glasper, 1995). Care should always be taken when oxygen is administered and this is outlined in Box 4.1.

Box 4.1. Safety precautions to be taken when oxygen is being used.

As oxygen is highly inflammable, these precautions must be followed to prevent accidental ignition (Campbell & Glasper, 1995):

- 'No Smoking' signs should be used
- All electrical appliances should be checked for safety
- Products containing petroleum or acetone should not be used
- Aerosol products should be avoided
- Synthetic material should be avoided to prevent static electricity
- Oxygen cylinders should be secured to prevent them from falling

---

As well as observing Michael, the pulse oximeter will warn the nurse of a drop in oxygen saturation levels. This is a measure of the percentage of oxygen bound to haemoglobin and should be 95–100% in healthy babies. The probe can cause burns to the skin, however, and should be repositioned 4 hourly to prevent this from occurring.

Nasopharyngeal suction may be required and this should be performed using the smallest cannula possible to avoid damage to the nasal tissues (Timby, 1996). The suction pressure should be kept low to reduce the risks of trauma to the tissues. Timby (1996) suggested that when wall-mounted suction units are used, the pressure should be 50–95 mmHg for infants.

As Michael is so breathless and unable to suck, fluids can be given via a nasogastric tube or via an IV infusion (see Profile 25, Caroline Davis). As babies' ribs do not slope downwards from the spine, the intercostal muscles are not used for breathing. Abdominal breathing is, therefore, normal (Campbell & Glasper, 1995). The nurse must ensure that Michael's breathing is not compromised if he is being fed by nasogastric tube. If this is the case, then an IV infusion must be commenced. It is important that Michael maintains an adequate fluid intake (Wong *et al.*, 1999) and his urinary output should be closely monitored.

If Michael was considered to be at high risk because of an underlying condition such as a congenital heart disorder and was found to have RSV, he might be commenced on Ribavarin, which is an antiviral drug. This is usually delivered into the oxygen headbox by means of a small-particle aerosol generator for 12–20 h (Wong *et al.*, 1999). There is evidence that Ribavarin can be toxic to both patients and staff, and care must, therefore, be taken if Michael is to be removed from the headbox. The drug should be discontinued first and several minutes should elapse between stopping the drug and removing Michael from the headbox (Wong *et al.*, 1999).

It is important to talk to Louise and Barry, who will no doubt be very anxious. James almost certainly has the same virus as Michael although at 2 years of age his airway is much larger and he can deal with the excess secretions. The parents must be warned that if James's secretions come into contact with Michael, he can be re-infected.

Michael should progress well and can return home within a few days.

References

Campbell, S., & Glasper, E. A. (eds) (1995). *Whaley and Wong's Children's Nursing.* London: Mosby.

Gould, D. (1997). A common ailment. *Nursing Times*, 93, 53–56.

Moules, T., & Ramsay, J. (1998). *The Textbook of Children's Nursing.* Cheltenham: Stanley Thornes.

Sadik, R., & Elliott, C. (1999). Respiration and circulation. In R. Hogston, & P. Simpson (eds), *Foundations of Nursing Practice* (167–215). London: Macmillan.

Timby, B. K. (1996). *Fundamental Skills & Concepts in Patient Care*, 6th edn. Philadelphia: Lippincott.

Wong, D. L., Hockenberry-Eaton, M., Wilson, D., Winkelstein, M. L., Ahmann, E., & DiVito-Thomas, P. A. (1999). *Whaley & Wong's Nursing Care of Infants and Children*, 6th edn. St Louis: Mosby.

Further reading

Burr, M. (1998, accessed 25 July 2000). Health Evidence Bulletins Wales: 3. Acute bronchiolitis and bronchitis
[http://www.uwcm.ac.uk/uwcm/lb/pep/respdis/chapter3.htm].

Everard, M. L. (1995). Bronchiolitis origins and optimal management. *Drugs*, 49, 885–896.

Klassen, T. P. (1997). Recent advances in the treatment of bronchiolitis and laryngitis. *Pediatric Clinics of North America*, 44, 249–261.

Martinez-Bianchi, V., Rejman-Peterson, M., & Graber, M. A. (1999, accessed 25 February 2000). Pediatrics: stridor and dyspnea
[http://www.vh.org/Providers/ClinRef/FPHandbook/Chapter10/20-10.htm].

Research Defence Society (1999, accessed 25 July 2000). Antibody therapy for bronchiolitis
[http://www.rds-online.org.uk/milestones/bronchio.htm].

Prematurity, respiratory distress and multiprofessional care

Joy Ward and Angela Jones

May Ling Brown is 3 months old and was born prematurely at 32 weeks gestation. At birth she clearly showed signs of respiratory distress, with Apgar scores of 5, 2 and 1. She subsequently spent 3 weeks being mechanically ventilated in the neonatal unit, where she was diagnosed as having bronchopulmonary dysplasia (BPD). During this time, May Ling has made good progress, but she still requires 0.3 litres oxygen via nasal cannulae to maintain oxygen saturations of 93–96%. Currently, May Ling is tolerating thickened oral feeds that the dietician had discussed with her mother Jackie and their named nurse.

Jackie lives with her partner Keiron, who is not the father of May Ling. May Ling's father, Chan, has no contact with Jackie or his daughter. Both Jackie and Keiron smoke and have no family living in the locality. Jackie is very keen to take May Ling home, and they have recently been allocated a two-bedroomed semidetached house in a low socio-economic district of the city. Neither Jackie nor Keiron are employed at present.

A discharge-planning meeting has been arranged to ensure a smooth transition into the community.

Question one: Explain who should be invited to attend the planning meeting.

10 minutes

Question two: Describe which statutory and voluntary organizations would be involved in May Ling's discharge.

10 minutes

Question three: Describe the types of equipment May Ling and her family might need for her discharge, stating where they would access it.

10 minutes

Question four: Using current research to support your answer, explain why early discharge on oxygen is the optimum situation for May Ling and her family.

20 minutes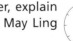

Time Allowance: **50 minutes**

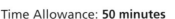

Answer to question one:
Explain who should be invited to attend the planning meeting.

Those asked to attend will include:

- Parents
- Social worker: advising about benefits and transportation to and from hospital appointments
- Community children's nurse: supporting, reassuring and teaching about the administration and safe provision of oxygen therapy. Teaching resuscitation skills. Nursing interventions such as oxygen saturation monitoring, assessing respiratory function and feeding regimens (Currie & Kotecha, 1997). Ascertaining and addressing any problems that may occur as a result of May Ling's disease pathology. Networking and coordinating other professionals. Continuity of care between home and hospital. Ensuring that the home is insured against fire
- Health visitor: checking and monitoring growth and developmental progress
- GP: coordinating medical aspects of care
- Consultant paediatrician: assessing pathological process progression
- Named nurse: continuity of care between hospital and home
- Dietician: informing about feed supplements and introducing a weaning diet in the future

Answer to question two:
Describe which statutory and voluntary organizations would be informed in May Ling's discharge.

- Physiotherapist: as May Ling has BPD she will need to receive chest physiotherapy on a regular basis
- Fire brigade: as oxygen supports combustion and both Jackie and Keiron smoke
- Insurance company: as oxygen in the property constitutes a risk
- A company to fit the oxygen equipment (safety pack and information provided), e.g. British Oxygen Cylinders Co., Boots. The family should be aware that public transport may not allow oxygen cylinders to be carried
- Premature baby support groups that may be running locally
- Other families who may have infants at home on oxygen
- Inform the local dispensing chemist who will supply equipment and replacement cylinders for the family

Answer to question three:

Describe the types of equipment May Ling and her family might need for her discharge, stating where they would access it.

- Portable oxygen cylinder (300 ml) supplied by their local chemist
- Oxygen flow meter, which can be obtained from the local health services
- Oxygen nasal cannulae, which may be supplied by the oxygen company, hospital, community nurses or GP health services
- GP: supplies prescription for tapes required for facial fixation and feed thickener
- Oxygen concentrator and pipes fitted by the oxygen equipment company
- Back-up cylinder holding 3400 litres oxygen or a generator in case of electricity failure

Answer to question four:
Using current research to support your answer, explain why early discharge on oxygen is the optimum situation for May Ling and her family.

The time that May Ling will remain oxygen-dependent is variable and can be affected by many factors. The indeterminable nature of her reliance on medical and nursing interventions could possibly indicate a prolonged period in an acute hospital setting. In the past, there would be no alternatives available to May Ling and her family, but as identified by Whiting (1997a) developments in community paediatric nursing have increased dramatically in the past decade. These developments have brought with them significant changes in the care available to infants with BPD (Currie & Kotecha, 1997).

The possibility of caring for May Ling within her home environment is reliant on appropriate planning and effective communication between all members of the multidisciplinary team in conjunction with Jackie and Keiron.

All professionals involved need to be aware of the emotional and physical demands made on parents when they take their babies home. Feelings of alarm and panic at their possible inability to cope with the enormous task of looking after a new baby, especially one requiring such intensive care and attention, may intimidate them, yet the desire to achieve some form of normality by returning home may restrict them from vocalizing any concerns.

Martin & Pridham (1992) stated that babies with BPD were generally unstable and difficult to feed. This may increase parents' anxiety levels and necessitate a great deal of additional help and assistance (Martin & Shaw, 1997). Despite potential difficulties, the provision of physical, practical and emotional support will ensure that the benefits of caring for May Ling at home will have long-lasting positive implications for all those involved. The benefits of caring for infants and children within their own homes have become more prevalent in the past decade. Hughes & Collins (1998) emphasized that prolonged periods of hospitalization could affect the emotional attachment between parents and their babies, which can be mainly overcome by home nursing care (Whiting, 1997b). Home care has also been identified as having positive financial implications for babies who require technological support (Youngblut et al., 1994), underpinning the continued drive to seek excellence in children's community nursing.

Children are being discharged into the community sicker and earlier than before. It is, therefore, important to acknowledge the need for continuous assessment of not only May Ling's needs, but also those of Jackie and Kieron, her primary carers.

Knafl & Deatrick (1990) devised a tool for assessing how well parents will cope with having a technologically dependent child at home. It involved three components:

- Assessment of social and cultural attitudes: how Jackie and Keiron react and cope with having an oxygen-dependent and premature infant
- How each member feels: their own way of identifying the important aspects of May Ling's condition and the impact that they perceive these might have on the family

- How each family member copes: how Jackie, Keiron and the extended family define the current situation and the degree of compromise each individual is prepared to make

Care planning should be a dynamic process that should adapt in partnership with the family as appropriate. This form of proactive practice will ensure that the road to independence for May Ling is not attained at the sacrifice of her parents' needs, and that the home environment is seen as a realistic choice for those children and families who deserve the benefits that primary health care can provide. In this case the benefits might include increased mother–child attachment, greater input in direct clinical care by the family and a greater say in the direction that May Ling's care will take. Other factors to consider are the reduced financial costs that regular hospital visits impose, improved feeding due to the reduced number of people involved in feeding May Ling as well as a reduced cross-infection risk. It is for all these reasons that community care for May Ling appears to provide an holistic solution to what might be a lengthy recovery period.

References

Currie, A. E., & Kotecha, S. (1997). Chronic lung disease of prematurity. *Care of the Critically Ill*, 13, 70–72.

Hughes, J., & Collins, S. P. (1998). Neonatal nursing in the community. *Paediatric Nursing*, 10, 18–20.

Knafl, K. A., & Deatrick, J. A. (1990). Family management style: concept analysis and development. *Journal of Pediatric Nursing*, 5, 4–14.

Martin, R. I., & Pridham, K. F. (1992). Early experiences of parents feeding their babies with BPD. *Neonatal Network: Journal of Neonatal Nursing*, 11, 23–29.

Martin, M., & Shaw, N. J. (1997). Feeding problems in infants and young children with chronic lung disease. *Journal of Human Nutrition and Dietetics*, 10, 271–275.

Whiting, M. (1997a). Forum of community children's nursing: a bright future? *Paediatric Nursing*, 9, 6–8.

Whiting, M. (1997b). Developing palliative care for children. *Paediatric Nursing*, 9, 3.

Youngblut, J. M., Brennan, P. F., & Swegart, L. A. (1994). Families with medically fragile children: an exploratory study. *Pediatric Nursing*, 20, 463–468.

Further reading

Audit Commission (1993). *Children First: A Study of Hospital Services for Children*. London: HMSO.

Coe, T., & Gallagher, A. (1999). Home is where the care is. *Nursing Times*, 95, 13–15.

Smith, S. (1999). Diana's legacy for life. *Nursing Times*, 95, 26–27.

Stephenson, C. (1999). Well-being of families with healthy and technology-assisted infants in the home: a comparative study. *Journal of Pediatric Nursing: Nursing Care of Children and Families*, 14, 164–176.

Neonate requiring stoma care

Leigh F. Caws

Nathan Simms, who was 4 months old, was causing concern to nursing/ medical staff and his parents due to a history of chronic constipation and difficulty in passing a meconium stool after birth. Nathan's abdomen was becoming noticeably distended and he appeared very agitated most of the time, drawing his legs up and crying inconsolably. His mother was attempting to breastfeed him, but both parties were becoming distressed and frustrated by the lack of success. Nathan was admitted to the hospital for investigation of a suspected bowel obstruction.

A barium enema revealed a very distended ganglionic portion of the colon and a rectal biopsy revealed an absence of ganglionic cells, which confirmed the diagnosis of Hirschsprung's disease.

Nathan weighed 5.7 kg so he would have to wait for complete surgical repair, which would only be effective when he weighed 8–10 kg. Meanwhile, palliative surgery would relieve the bowel obstruction by fashioning a temporary colostomy with the most distal section of normal bowel (Figure 6.1).

Following an uneventful pregnancy, Mr and Mrs Simms were shocked by the news of their firstborn child. This threw them into a state of confusion, as Mrs Simms was a barrister and had employed a nanny as she was planning to return to work within the next 2 weeks. However, they were keen to accompany Nathan on his transferral to the regional childrens' surgical unit 20 miles away. He was transferred in a portable incubator with a peripheral IV line and nasogastric tube *in situ* to stabilize his condition.

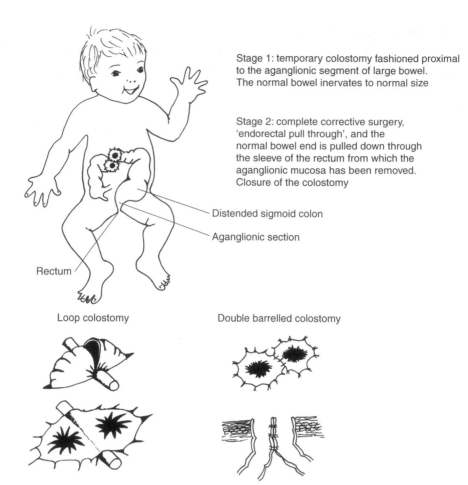

Stage 1: temporary colostomy fashioned proximal to the aganglionic segment of large bowel. The normal bowel inervates to normal size

Stage 2: complete corrective surgery, 'endorectal pull through', and the normal bowel end is pulled down through the sleeve of the rectum from which the aganglionic mucosa has been removed. Closure of the colostomy

Distended sigmoid colon

Aganglionic section

Rectum

Loop colostomy

Double barrelled colostomy

Figure 6.1. Hirshsprung's disease and the colostomy function.

Question one: Giving explanations for interventions, devise a teaching plan for Nathan's parents and the nanny that will allow them to provide stoma care for him.

1 hour

Time Allocation: **1 hour**

Answer to question one:
Giving explanations for interventions, devise a teaching plan for Nathan's parents and the nanny that will allow them to provide stoma care for him.

The nursing objectives that needed to be achieved to ensure a successful teaching plan for the parents and nanny were to:

- Minimize barriers to learning
- Encourage family involvement, including other carers such as grandparents and the nanny
- Support and guide parents, making appropriate specialist referrals
- Ensure a clear understanding of the purpose and function of Nathan's colostomy

The teaching plan should be prepared by breaking down the skills and knowledge required to learn into well-defined parts to prevent repetition and confusion. Learning outcomes need to be clear and concise, giving the parents the rationale for the skills learned to improve understanding and compliance. It is important to remember that parents are often frightened, upset and repulsed at the first sight of the stoma.

Moules & Ramsey (1999) highlighted concerns that parents express about their child's colostomy, such as:

- Will I hurt him when I change the bag?
- Can he have a bath?
- How often do I change the bag?
- How will I manage if I want to go out?
- Can he go swimming?
- What will people say?
- Will it smell?
- Will people tell that he has a colostomy?

Colostomy and its function

Goals:

- To ensure an understanding of Hirschsprung's disease and the purpose of the colostomy
- To differentiate between colostomy, ileostomy and urostomy to avoid confusion when meeting other children/families with stomas

Actions:

- According to their previous knowledge, define and explain Hirschsprung's disease clearly as a defect that occurs in the colon where nerve cells called ganglion nerves are absent and faeces cannot pass through the abnormal section of gut leading to chronic constipation and colic type pain
- Define a 'temporary' colostomy as an opening made into the large intestine (colon) to externalize it onto the abdomen to pass faeces involuntarily into a bag placed via the stoma

- Differentiate between colostomy, ileostomy and urostomy. Explain that an ileostomy is essentially the same as a colostomy but the small intestine (ileum) is externalized instead and fashioned as more of a spout as the faecal waste is more liquid in nature
- Briefly mention that a urostomy is an opening made to divert urine from the bladder using a piece of intestine to fashion a stoma

Equipment and appliances

Goals:

- To explain the differences and uses of stoma care appliances
- To provide an appliance for Nathan that is well fitting, comfortable, non-irritating and odour-proof with sufficient bag capacity

Actions:
See Table 6.1.

Table 6.1. Actions and explanations.

Action	Explanation
Show Mr and Mrs Simms and the nanny the 'one-piece' ostomy bag, which is a simple bag that can be closed or non-drainable for a colostomy. The stoma fits into the hole and the self-adhesive wafer sticks onto the skin around the stoma	These types of ostomy bags are fixed around the stoma by a self-adhesive wafer or skin protector with a hole cut into it to allow faecal drainage and prevent leakage for faecal waste which contains enzymes that break down skin at contact. The advantage of this is that the whole bag can be removed and discarded with its contents, leaving the protective base-plate on the skin
Demonstrate the use of a 'two-piece' bag, which has a base-plate that fits around the stoma with separate bags attached to the base-plate	This more rigid appliance can cause problems because there is a limited surface area on which to apply the base-plate and there can be difficulty in moulding it to the infant's abdomen (Fitzpatrick, 1996). This may be useful if faecal waste is thin, as this is likely to be the case due to the faster passage of breast milk through the gut. When weaning is established, the faeces become more solid with a colostomy as some of the liquid is absorbed through the healthy part of the colon. A drainable appliance is preferable on infants to avoid frequent changing (Fitzpatrick, 1996)
'Drainable bags' could be used while Nathan is breastfed until weaning is well established. A clip secures the base of the bag and is removed for emptying purposes. The clip might be uncomfortable against Nathan's body and, therefore, it could be unsuitable	A snug fit of the stoma is important to prevent faecal leakage and odour. The bag ring must not touch the sides of the stoma as this might cause irritation, abrasions and cuts. After the initial trauma of the surgery, the stoma might become smaller due to the reduction of swelling with time (Parry, 1998)
Select or fashion the correct aperture size and shape for the stoma by using the measuring ring provided by the manufacturer, which can be cut accordingly	

Goal:

- To teach the parents and other carers, e.g. nanny, how to prepare, empty and change the colostomy appliance

Action:
See Table 6.2.

Table 6.2. Actions and explanations.

Action	Explanation
On average the appliance should be changed every 2–3 days (Fitzpatrick, 1996) if it is a two-piece or drainable pouch and emptied when necessary	To minimize trauma to the skin and stoma
Gather the following equipment: - Plastic gloves (optional for parents) - Towel - Warm water (mild soap – optional) - Stoma bag with clamp and other fittings - Clean gauze squares - Nappy bucket/plastic bag to hand - Stoma barrier creams, wafers, paste and powder - Scissors	It is important to be well organized to avoid leaving Nathan and to run the risk of creating an unpleasant mess. Nurses must wear gloves to prevent cross-infection. Only water or mild soap are used to reduce skin dryness. The stoma nurse will measure the size of the stoma for the correct appliance. Gauze is placed over the stoma to act as a wick while cleaning the site (Ashwill and Droske, 1997). A nappy bucket is hygienic and easy to dispose of. Stoma barrier creams, etc. protect the skin around the stoma site. Scissors cut the aperture in ostomy bag
The procedure to be taught: - If the appliance is drainable, empty the bag into a disposable pot and dispose of the soiled bag, etc. by wrapping it in newspaper and placing it in a plastic bag for bin disposal - Never flush ostomy bags down the toilet, for this can block them! - Gently remove the existing appliance - If a paste or cement has been used to adhere the previous bag to the skin, a special solvent should be applied with a cotton bud before removal	Proper disposal of the bag will prevent cross-infection and contamination. The bags must be removed gently to minimize skin and stoma trauma by supporting the skin with one hand and pulling the appliance with the other (NASPCS, 1993; Fitzpatrick, 1996)
Clean the stoma area gently using warm water and a sponge/gauze. If soap is used, choose a mild one and rinse off well. Some residue left by the sticking plaster may build up on the skin; this is harmless and may be left. Products for removing these may be used cautiously	Rubbing the stoma/skin is an abrasive action. Soap dries the skin and may cause irritation. Sticky tape will not have been used on Nathan to minimize excoriation. These products often sting and should never be used if the skin is sore (NASPCS, 1993)
Nathan may benefit from a bath at this point if convenient. Dry the skin thoroughly and apply gauze swabs over the stoma	This is a time for bath play, bonding interaction and freedom from appliances (Fitzpatrick, 1996). A dry skin will ensure good adhesion of the appliance and the gauze will mop up faecal leakage while drying Nathan

Table 6.2. – *continued*

Action	Explanation
A skin barrier may be applied to the area around the stoma following the manufacturer's instructions before attachment of the ostomy appliance. This may come as a powder, spray, cream, liquid or invisible skin. Finally, the correct-sized appliance can be adhered to the stoma Tape should never be used to reinforce a leaking appliance (Fitzpatrick, 1996)	A skin barrier also helps to prevent skin excoriation, but Fitzpatrick (1996) advised that one use a 'patch test' with the chosen product 24 h before use to ensure that an allergic reaction does not occur around the stoma site. Leakage of faecal material onto the skin causes soreness very quickly on neonatal skin as babies have a thinner and more delicate skin than have older children and adults
When emptying the colostomy bag between changes, the inside of the pouch can be rinsed with 60 ml tap water. This reduces odour and an unpleasant appearance of the bag (Ashwill and Droske, 1997)	

Diet and nutrition

Goal:

- To ensure that Nathan's parents and other carers appropriate to him have a full understanding of his nutritional needs to so that he can fulfil his growth potential

Action:
See Table 6.3.

Table 6.3. Actions and explanations.

Action	Explanation
Nathan can be breastfed normally and should his mother wish to transfer him onto mixed feeding or just formula milk feeds before starting work, she may do so	Breastfeeding for as long as possible will provide Nathan with an enhanced immune system and the correct balance of nutrients that are readily absorbed by the infant (DHSS, 1988)
Weaning Nathan can be commenced at 4–6 months of age as normal (DoH, 1994), but low-residue foods might be preferable initially to prevent faecal waste from the colostomy becoming too liquid	It is important to give Nathan a normal diet conducive to his physical and psychosocial development (see Profile 11, Patrick Cooper). Weaning foods will generally make the stool less liquid, although parents need to experiment with different foods in the diet to determine their effects on consistency
Extra fluids such as cooled boiled water and dilute fruit juice should be given during hot weather, with a fever or with bouts of diarrhoea (NASPCS, 1993)	Nathan is at risk of rapid onset of dehydration under these conditions due to the fast metabolic rate of neonates and in his case the reduced colonic absorption (Fitzpatrick, 1996)

Complications

Goal:

- To reduce anxiety, explain to the family and nanny how to anticipate and detect at an early stage problems that might arise with the colostomy and teach them how to deal with these

Action:
See Table 6.4.

Table 6.4. Actions and explanations.

Action	Explanation
Explain to the parents and nanny what to do in the event of the following complications:	
• Surface bleeding due to superficial trauma	Check that Nathan is not scratching the stoma site. If so, reapply a new appliance and place cotton mittens on his hands. Make sure that the ostomy appliance is not irritating the stoma and reapply as necessary. There is no cause for alarm
• Bleeding from inside the stoma or ribbon-like stools (Moules and Ramsey, 1999)	Report to the GP; this should not occur
• Prolapse of the stoma can occur in a colostomy and this may be frightening. It can be caused by a bout of coughing or crying (NASPCS, 1993)	This is due to an increase in intra-abdominal pressure created by activities such as coughing. No immediate action is required so long as the stoma remains pink-red, looks healthy, continues to function and there is no sign of pain, i.e. undue crying, grimacing, drawing up of the legs. The prolapse usually reduces at nighttime or during sleep (Fitzpatrick, 1996). If it persists contact the GP
• Diarrhoea, which may be due to an infection (viral or bacterial) or certain foods or medications such as antibiotics	One should expect a liquid to semisolid stool while breastfeeding, which should thicken slightly with formula feeds and a weaning diet. If loss is excessive and the baby is unwell, contact the GP and give extra clear fluids
• Constipation is possible, but unusual in infancy	If this occurs, give Nathan fruit juices if weaned. Continue breastfeeding if appropriate
• Odour and excessive flatus	This should not be too problematic especially if breastfed. If anything it is less offensive than defecating conventionally into a nappy. Odour may be worse with certain types of foods used for weaning

Support mechanisms

Goals:

- Highlight a range of support mechanisms
- Explore a few useful tips to make family life easier

Actions:
See Table 6.5.

Table 6.5. Actions and explanations.

Action	Explanation
Introduce the family to the stoma care nurse	Such a nurse is usually in a hospital and will always give help, teaching and advice during the in-patient period as well as at home. The nurse is a specialist in the field of stoma care and offers advice on equipment
Health visitor support	Knows the local stoma care facilities and performs regular developmental assessments and baby weights. Advises on feeding practices and problems
GP	Prescribes ostomy appliances weekly to monthly, which can be collected at the local pharmacy or delivered to the home by post. These should be stored out of direct sunlight and away from heat to avoid spoilage. Provides help for general health issues for Nathan
Parents may wish to contact the National Advisory Service for Parents of Children with a Stoma (NASPCS)	Provides leaflets, advice, support, can put the family in contact with other families who have children/infants with stomas and provides information on ostomy care and diseases related to ostomies
May wish to register with the British Colostomy Association	As above, but focuses on older children and adults
Answer any trouble shooting questions such as:	
• Can I take my baby swimming?	Yes, patterned costumes may disguise the bag (no diving, though, for which Nathan is far too young)
• Can we go abroad or on holiday?	Yes, there are travel kits suggested in the NASPCS booklet. Take a good supply of appliances and skin barriers, etc. Contact the GP first and take out medical insurance

Throughout the teaching programme, which will vary in duration according to the parents' and nanny's acceptance of the situation and personal learning curve, it is important to emphasize that normal family life is the ultimate goal. Parents often have feelings of grief due to the loss of their 'perfect baby' and guilt that something they have done wrong during the pregnancy caused the defect (Fitzpatrick, 1996). Reassurance is essential, particularly as the problem can be rectified with relative ease between 6–12 months of age. New parenthood is challenging, but the added dimension of a baby which has a colostomy and requiring further surgery means that stresses can be immense.

References

Ashwill, J. W. and Droske, S. C. (1997). *Nursing Care of Children: Principles and Practice.* Philadelphia: W. B. Saunders.

Department of Health (DoH) (1994). *Weaning and the Weaning Diet.* Report on Health and Social Subjects no. 45. London: HMSO.

Department of Health and Social Security (DHSS) (1988). *Present Day Practice in Infant Feeding.* Third Report. Report on Health and Social Subjects no. 32. London: HMSO.

Fitzpatrick, G. (1996). The child with a stoma. In C. Myers (ed.), *Stoma Care Nursing* (180–202). London: Arnold.

Moules, T., & Ramsey, J. (1999). *The Textbook of Children's Nursing.* Cheltenham: Stanley Thornes.

National Advisory Service for Parents of Children with a Stoma (NASPCS) (1993). *Our Special Children: A Practical Guide to Stoma Care in Babies and Young Children.* High Wycombe: CliniMed.

Parry, A. (1998). Stoma care in the neonates: improving practice. *Journal of Neonatal Nursing,* 4, 8–11.

Infant who is failing to thrive

Leigh F. Caws

Lo Chan is 6 months old and has Down's syndrome. He was born in the UK after his parents arrived from China 7 months ago. Mr Chan is a physics student at the local university where he secured a place on a degree course before the family's arrival in the country. Separation from the extended family is proving stressful and difficult, particularly for his wife as there is no support or guidance for her with the baby. The couple are Taoist and Mr Chan has managed to contact other Chinese students in the city and is slowly making friends through his studies. However, Mrs Chan appears to be becoming more socially isolated and is struggling to learn English.

Ellen, the health visitor visits the family home, which is a rented bedsit in a three-bedroomed house near the university, once a fortnight as she is concerned about the baby's poor weight gain. Lo was born at 36 weeks' gestation and weighed 2.5 kg, at 2 months old he weighed 4.5 kg and currently weighs 5.8 kg. He is 68 cm long and his head circumference is 45 cm.

Mrs Chan continues to breastfeed her child but, as yet, has not introduced weaning foods. He looks malnourished and underweight and the health visitor is very concerned about the general health and welfare of both mother and baby. Lo developed gastro-enteritis 3 days ago and has not passed urine for 24 h. The health visitor feels that clinically he appears 10% dehydrated and immediately takes them both to the paediatric department at the local hospital.

Question one: Justify the nursing assessment of Lo in relation to his hydration status.

30 minutes

Question two: Rationalize the main nursing interventions for the family, considerate of their cultural and religious beliefs.

1 hour

Time Allowance: **1 hour 30 minutes**

Answer to question one:
Justify the nursing assessment of Lo in relation to his hydration status.

Lo is likely to be experiencing isotonic (serum sodium 135–141 mmol l^{-1}) dehydration. This is because gastro-enteritis tends to lead to a loss of water and electrolytes in about the same proportions as they exist in the body. Hydration is usually assessed in terms of percentage dehydration related to symptoms and as Lo is ~10% dehydrated and is bordering on the moderate-to-severe classification with the resulting clinical features shown in Table 7.1.

Table 7.1. Guide to the assessment of dehydration of infants (adapted from Betz *et al.*, 1994).

	Mild dehydration	Moderate	Severe
Loss of body weight (%)	< 5	5–10	10
Skin colour	pale	dusky	mottled/dark circles around eyes
Skin turgor	decreased	moderately decreased	markedly decreased
Urine output	decreased	oliguria	oliguria/anuria
Thirst	slight	moderate	intense
Tears	present	decreased	absent
Mucous membranes	dry or sticky	very dry	parched/absence of tears
BP	normal	normal or slightly above or below normal	low
Pulse	normal or tachycardia	tachycardia	increased tachycardia and thready pulse
Anterior fontanelles	level or flat	slightly sunken	sunken/suture lines may be prominent

To make a full nursing assessment of Lo's hydration status, his aural temperature would have to be taken due to the likelihood of a pyrexia derived from the gastro-enteritis. This increases fluid requirements and metabolic rate, which may ultimately lead to a metabolic acidosis, initially compensated for by tachypnoea.

His BP may be decreased in severe dehydration, but this is a late sign of shock as infants have an effective compensatory mechanism to maintain adequate cardiac output. Therefore, changes in heart rate, pulse and skin colour are more reliable indicators of shock (Hazinski, 1999).

Weighing Lo's nappies would confirm a diminished urinary output of < 1–2 ml kg^{-1} h^{-1} (in Lo's case this would be < 11.6 ml h^{-1}) and a specific gravity > 1.020 might indicate dehydration, although the presence of glucose or protein in the urine would interfere with the parameter. In reality, urine output may be difficult to assess accurately by nappy weight due to the diarrhoea caused by the gastro-enteritis. It may be necessary to catheterize the baby if he is severely compromised to ascertain renal function. On dipstick urine testing, one would expect to see positive readings for ketones due to the fat catabolism of a starving baby.

Lo's stools and vomitus should be observed for consistency, type, frequency and quantity. His weight would be recorded for a baseline reading on admission, then daily until he was rehydrated. Weight may not be a good indicator for the degree of dehydration in this case as Lo has a history of poor weight gain. His birth weight was just over the 25th centile and by 2 months of age it had fallen to between the 0.4 and 2nd centiles, this already showing clear signs of failure to thrive. His weight on admission was around the 2nd centile, but this would be difficult to assess accurately due to the dehydration.

The nurse would also observe Lo for signs of hyponatraemia (serum sodium of < 135 mmol l^{-1}) in the form of irritability, tachycardia, cold clammy skin, abdominal and leg cramps that might be difficult to assess in this age group. The doctor would also need assistance to take venous blood samples for urea and electrolyte levels to confirm imbalances.

Hypokalaemia (serum potassium of < 3.5 mmol l^{-1}) would cause cardiac arrhythmias, tachycardia or bradycardia best observed for by using a cardiac monitor.

Finally, Lo would probably be irritable and lethargic and may have a high pitched and weak cry due to cerebral irritation caused by dehydration. If this state persists, then he will probably also experience seizures. One would also expect a low blood glucose (3–4 mmol l^{-1}) from a heel prick blood sample as a result of reduced carbohydrate intake and lactose lost in the diarrhoea.

Answer to question two:
Rationalize the main nursing interventions for the family, considerate of their cultural and religious beliefs.

Communication

Talking to Mr Chan should be relatively easy as he is attending a course at the local university and, therefore, probably has a reasonable command of English. Detailed explanations of the nursing care, treatment and investigations should be provided when he is present, so that he can interpret this for his wife and so reduce her anxiety. Nursing care can also be delivered through a family-centred care philosophy using the 'Partnership in Care' model (Casey, 1988). This will enable the multidisciplinary team to meet the specific needs of the family. The Taoist philosophy is to find 'the way' or 'Tao', which is achieved through following the way of Nature (Shih, 1996). This may account for the mother's commitment to breastfeeding and possible reluctance to wean despite his poor weight gain. Some Taoist people believe in a cold 'Yin' energy and a hot 'Yang', which should be balanced to produce harmony for the 'Chi' (energy or spirit of one's body). If there is an excess of Yin, the person may be prone to infections and gastric problems, for example, and an excess of Yang could lead to dehydration, fever and irritability (Chan, 1995), symptoms which Lo is exhibiting.

It is essential to explain the importance of thorough hand washing and the principles of infection control while Lo's diarrhoea and vomiting persists, and he is being nursed in a cubicle.

Hydration

Lo requires initial IV replacement of the circulating blood volume. According to Insley (1996), this is normally achieved through the use of plasma or 0.9% sodium chloride at 20 ml kg^{-1} of body weight over 1–2 h, which would amount to 116 ml over 2 h for Lo. Maintenance IV therapy should be 0.18% sodium chloride in 4% dextrose at up to 100 ml kg^{-1} in 24 h (Insley, 1996). Based on this calculation, Lo would require 580 ml in 24 h (24–25 ml h^{-1}). IV tubing and solutions should be changed daily to prevent bacterial colonization (Moules and Ramsey, 1998) and reduce the risk of septicaemia. The cannula should be secured with a sterile dressing as the use of non-sterile adhesive tape can lead to an increased risk of contamination (Oldman, 1991), and the site should be observed 2–4 hourly for signs of inflammation and phlebitis. If the cannulated limb needs to be immobilized, the correctly sized splint should be applied, and pressure points protected and inspected frequently. The use of wooden tongue depressors wrapped in gauze and sponge for splinting is contraindicated due to the high risk of systemic infection (Editorial, 1996). Adverse effects from IV therapy should be reported to the doctor immediately and the cannula should be resited. The nurse should be particularly vigilant about the invasive nature of IV therapy as those of Chinese extraction are very sensitive to intrusive procedures (Shih, 1996).

Diet needs to be re-established so that Lo can begin to gain weight to the expected level. This would normally be calculated using the following guidelines:

- Weight loss of up to 10% of an infant's birth weight is to be expected by day 3 (this can be greater in the preterm infant)
- 200 g per week weight gain for the first 3 months
- 150 g per week weight gain for the second 3 months
- 100 g per week weight gain for the third 3 months
- 50–75g per week weight gain for the fourth 3 months (Thompson, 1998)

However, Lo was preterm (born before 37 weeks gestation) and classified as low birth weight (LBW; < 2.5 kg). Plotting his weight on the boy's growth foundation chart (1994) reveals his growth status:

- Birth weight 2.5 kg: just above the 25th centile
- At 2 months of age 4.5 kg: between 0.4th and 2nd centile
- At 5 months of age 5.8 kg (dehydrated) at 2nd centile

His expected weight around the 25th centile (which should approximate to his growth curve) should be ~6.6 kg based on growth curves for British infants; however, this is not considerate of Chinese growth and stature.

While Lo is still suffering from gastro-enteritis, breastfeeding may continue, but for this to be more successful, a dietary assessment of the mother is essential. This would allow the nursing staff to advise her on nutrient and fluid requirements to improve the quality of her milk and to prevent her state of malnourishment from worsening. Energy requirements during lactation should be increased according to the recommendations detailed in Table 7.2 (DoH, 1991).

Table 7.2. COMA recommendations on dietary references for the lactating woman.

Stage of lactation (months)	Extra kcal
0–1	450
1–2	530
2–3	570
3–6	480
> 6	240

Foods should be chosen from milk and dairy foods, although these foods do not feature significantly in the Chinese diet of meat, fish, soya, bread, rice, other cereals, fruit and vegetables. One explanation for this is that many Chinese people suffer from lactose intolerance.

An extra 11 g protein is also required (DoH, 1991), a day that can be met by increasing these food groups. Mrs Chan should be advised to drink to satisfy her thirst, explaining that dark or strong-smelling urine indicates the need to drink more. It is thought that fluctuations in fluid intake should not affect milk production (Dusdieker *et al.*, 1985). Breastfeeding would also be observed to ensure the infant had an effective technique particularly as Lo might experience feeding difficulties due to a large protruding tongue and a narrow, high arched palate, which are clinical features of Down's syndrome (Ashwill and Droske, 1997). If vomiting persists and breast milk is not tolerated initially, Mrs Chan could be encouraged and assisted to express and freeze her milk so that feeding may resume in due course. Meanwhile, the baby could be commenced on an oral rehydration solution. Mrs Chan might prefer her son to have a rice-based oral rehydration solution with glucose that has proven effective and reduced hospital admission time (Wall *et al.*, 1997).

Once vomiting and diarrhoea have ceased and breastfeeding is well established, weaning foods should be introduced to boost Lo's energy and iron intake. This is important as premature infants are usually born with reduced iron and zinc stores (NDC, 1995), which, even in full-term infants, are depleted by 6 months of age. The DoH COMA Report on Weaning and the Weaning Diet (1994) advises that the majority of infants should not be given solid foods before 4 months of age. However, one must exercise caution with this directive as Lo was premature and gastrointestinal maturation might be slightly delayed in relation to chronological age as weaning is not recommended before 16 weeks post-delivery or before the premature infant is 5 kg (Lawson, 1991). In either case, Lo is well within the recommended guidelines for safe introduction of solid food. It is important to introduce solids into Lo's diet as soon as possible not only to promote weight gain and growth, but also to enhance chewing and biting skills, which assist mouth/tongue coordination in preparation for speech, stimulate tooth eruption and prevent rejection of different tastes and textures during the preschool years.

Weaning can be initiated in hospital until a steady weight gain is evident and Mrs Chan feels confident enough to provide for Lo's care. Mr and Mrs Chan would be taught about providing a healthy diet for their baby. The benefits of dairy produce, which can be introduced from 6 months of age to ensure adequate calcium intake for bone growth, might need to be highlighted. The risk of hypernatraemia and resulting dehydration when adding salt to Lo's food should be explained to the parents as the Chinese diet tends to be high in salt (Thompson, 1998). Manufactured first-stage weaning foods may be too expensive for the family budget, although convenient and possibly more hygienic due to the limited cooking facilities of a bedsit. Modifying their own foods to provide pureed vegetables, stewed non-citrus fruits, meats, pulses and gluten-free cereals such as baby rice and cooked ground maize might be an option, but food hygiene and storage needs careful explanation to prevent further episodes of gastro-enteritis. Second-stage weaning foods that can be introduced from 6 months of age should include foods from all food groups including dairy produce and cereals containing gluten, which are mashed, lumpy or finger foods. The parents should be advised to start with small amounts of three-to-four teaspoons two or three times a day, gradually increasing the quantity and introducing new foods. It should be emphasized that added sugar should be avoided or used very sparingly to prevent sweet food preference, dental decay and obesity.

It is vitally important to ensure that the family has the support, nutritional advice and food hygiene information from the health visitor on a weekly basis, including weekly weights, preferably at the baby clinic. They will be asked to bring Lo to the hospital for an outpatient appointment in a few week's time and he will need a physiotherapy and developmental assessment due to his Down's syndrome. The family may benefit from contact with The Down's Syndrome Association to gain a clearer understanding of what the future may hold for them and resources available while they are in the UK.

References

Ashwill, J. W., & Droske, S. C. (1997). *Nursing Care of Children: Principles and Practice*. Philadelphia: W. B. Saunders.

Betz, C. L., Hunsberger, M. M., & Wright, S. (1994). *Family Centred Nursing Care of Children*, 2nd edn. Philadelphia: W. B. Saunders.

Casey, A. (1988). A partnership with child and family. *Senior Nurse*, 18, 8–9.

Chan, J. Y. K (1995). Dietary beliefs of Chinese patients. *Nursing Standard*, 9, 30–34.

Department of Health (1991). *Dietary Reference Values: A Guide*. London: HMSO.

Department of Health (1994). *Weaning and the Weaning Diet*. Report on Health and Social Subjects no. 45. London: HMSO.

Dusdieker, L. B., Booth, B. M., Stumbo, P. J., & Waterston, A. J. R. (1985). Effect of supplementary fluids on human milk production. *Journal of Paediatrics*, 106, 207–211.

Editorial (1996). Stop using tongue depressors as splints. *Paediatric Nursing*, 8, 4.

Growth Foundation Chart (1994). *Boys Four-in-One Growth Chart*. London: CGF.

Hazinski, M. F. (1999). *Nursing Care of the Critically Ill Child*. London: Mosby.

Insley, J. (1996). *A Paediatric Vade-Mecum*. London: Lloyd-Luke.

Lawson, M. (1994). Low birth weight infants. In V. Shaw, & M. Lawson (eds), *Clinical Paediatric Dietetics* (51–60). Oxford: Blackwells.

Moules, T., & Ramsey, J. (1998). *The Textbook of Children's Nursing*. Cheltenham: Stanley Thornes.

National Dairy Council (1995). *Nutrition of Infants and Children*. Fact File 2. London: NDC.

Oldman, P. (1991). A sticky situation; microbiological study of adhesive tape used to secure intravenous cannulae. *Professional Nurse*, 6, 265–269.

Shih, F. J. (1996). Psycho-social concepts related to Chinese patients' perceptions of health, illness and person: issues of conceptual clarity, *Accident and Emergency Nursing*, 4, 208–215.

Thompson, J. M. (1998). *Nutritional Requirements of Infants and Young Children: Practical Guidelines*. Oxford: Blackwells.

Wall, C. R., Swanson, C. E., & Cleghorn G. (1997). Re-hydration in infants with gastro-enteritis. *Journal of Gastroenterology*, 12, 24–28.

Useful information

Down's Syndrome Association, 155 Mitcham Road, London SW17 9PG, UK; tel.: 020 8682 4001; http://www.downs-syndrome.org.uk/

Dysplasia of the hip and Gallows traction

Jane McConochie

Samantha was the firstborn child of John and Julia. She was born at 39 weeks gestation following an elective Caesarean section for an extended breech.

A postnatal examination revealed that her right leg tended to move only to the right and that the hip remained naturally in a fixed position, although it was possible to straighten the leg.

Julia remained concerned about Samantha's right leg and mentioned it to the health visitor, Susan, when she next visited the family. On examination, Susan thought that the right leg was possibly shorter than the left leg and recommended that Julia made an appointment to see her GP.

On examination the GP found that not only was there possible shortening of the right leg, but also that there was reduction in the muscle covering the thigh of the affected leg. Samantha was now 3 months old and the GP felt that referral to an orthopaedic consultant was essential.

Samantha was seen by the orthopaedic consultant whose examination revealed that the thigh creases were asymmetric and that there was a gross restriction of movement when the right hip was abducted. There was also evidence of plagiocephaly (distortion of the shape of the skull) secondary to preferential left sided lying. Ultrasound examination suggested that the right hip was not developing normally and that the head of the femur showed only a small ossific nucleus (becoming bone). X-ray confirmed the presence of the small ossific nucleus on the right side with evidence of acetabular dysplasia with possible subluxation of the leg. This confirmed the diagnosis of developmental dysplasia of the hip (DDH) (formerly known as congenital dislocation of the hip, CDH).

Owing to her age and the result of the X-rays, the consultant explained that the best course of treatment would be for Samantha to be admitted to the children's ward for 1 week of Gallows traction and an arthrogram. It might then be possible to carry out a closed reduction of the hip and apply a plaster hip spica rather than an internal reduction and fixation of the hip.

When 7 months old, Samantha was admitted to hospital for the above treatment to be carried out. The hip was successfully reduced and a plaster hip spica applied.

Question one: Explain the nursing care that Samantha should receive while on Gallows traction.

45 minutes

Time Allowance: **45 minutes**

Answer to question one:

Explain the nursing care that Samantha should receive while on Gallows traction.

When Samantha is on Gallows traction, her legs are suspended in the air and her body provides the counterweight. It should, therefore, be possible to slide a hand under her bottom (Carter & Dearmun, 1995). The skin traction, usually adhesive, is bandaged into place (Figure 8.1).

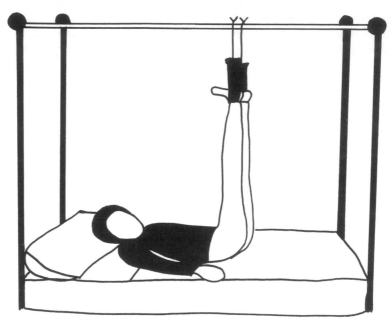

Figure 8.1. Gallows traction. Buttocks must be kept clear of the bed.

While on traction, a neurovascular assessment should be made regularly to ensure that there is no impairment (Strycula, 1994). This includes regularly checking the pulses, capillary refill time, colour and warmth of Samantha's feet (see Profile 25, Caroline Davis).

Her bandages should be removed daily to check skin integrity. This will also be a time to assess that the traction itself is not peeling off Samantha's legs. Care must be taken to ensure that Samantha's traction is level and that one leg is not raised higher than the other and that the knots in the rope are secure (Timby, 1996). Samantha should have enough room under the traction to move her feet and ankles (Campbell & Glasper, 1995). Checking pressure areas is important, particularly Samantha's shoulders and the back of her head, to identify if the areas are red or sore. Samantha should be encouraged to move around in the cot. The nurses and family should be careful to keep the sheets under Samantha crumb and wrinkle free and to avoid pulling the sheets from under Samantha, which could cause friction or shearing injury. A child's pressure sore risk assessment could be undertaken using a recognized tool such as that developed by Bedi (1993).

Hygiene is essential and John and Julia should be encouraged to wash and dress Samantha with assistance being given as required (Casey, 1988; Darbyshire, 1994). Samantha's nappies should be changed frequently to prevent seepage of urine, which can be difficult to prevent while she is suspended on traction. Samantha's bowels should be monitored to identify if she is becoming constipated. This can be prevented by encouraging mobility, ensuring an adequate fluid intake of 100 ml kg^{-1} day^{-1} (Moules & Ramsay, 1998) and by providing a healthy balanced diet appropriate to her age.

The immobility of traction might cause Samantha's appetite to fluctuate. It is important to ensure that she receives a balanced diet and, while finger food is to be encouraged, she should always be supervised when eating to prevent choking. When Samantha is offered a bottle feed, an arm can be placed under her shoulders to raise her head to a more appropriate feeding position. When solids are being offered, it should be in small quantities offered frequently.

Owing to her abnormal body positioning, Samantha may not sleep for as long as usual. She is using less energy due to limited mobility and, therefore, is not as tired as normal. Providing plenty of stimulation and play activities when she is awake may help this situation.

Temperature, pulse and respiration rate should be monitored daily. If there is an increase in any of these vital signs, it may indicate a chest infection, in which case the doctor should be informed and antibiotics might be prescribed. These observations should then be recorded 4 hourly. It is important to reassure and assist Julia and John so that they can care for Samantha. It can be very daunting to look after someone on traction for the first time.

References

Bedi, A. (1993). A tool to fill the gap: developing a wound risk assessment chart for children. *Professional Nurse*, 9, 112–118.

Campbell, S., & Glasper, E. A. (eds) (1995). *Whaley and Wong's Children's Nursing*. London: Mosby.

Carter, B., & Dearmun, A. K. (eds) (1995). *Child Health Care Nursing*. Oxford: Blackwells.

Casey, A. (1988). A partnership with child and family. *Senior Nurse*, 18, 8–9.

Darbyshire, P. (1994). *Living with a Sick Child in Hospital: The Experiences of Parents and Nurses*. London: Chapman & Hall.

Moules, T., & Ramsay, J. (1998). *The Textbook of Children's Nursing*. Cheltenham: Stanley Thornes.

Strycula, L. (1994). Traction basics: Part IV. Traction for lower extremities. *Orthopaedic Nursing*, 13, 59–68.

Timby, B. K. (1996). *Fundamental Skills & Concepts in Patient Care*, 6th edn. Philadelphia: Lippincott.

Further reading

Anon. (n.d., accessed 25 July 2000). Developmental dysplasia of the hip [http://onhealth.com/conditions/resource/conditions/item,52105.as].

Anon. (n.d., accessed 25 July 2000). The management of fractures of the femur [http://www.jr2.ox.ac.uk/nds/Simple-Surgery/Procedures/Femoralfrac].

Shoppee, K. (1992). Developmental dysplasia of the hip. *Orthopaedic Nursing*, 11, 30–36.

Waterlow, J. (1997). Pressure sore risk assessment in children. *Paediatric Nursing*, 9, 21–24.

Head injury

Christine Ward

Jason is 18 months old and is the only child of Jess and Ian King. He is a lively toddler with endless amounts of energy.

It was early one morning when Jason was helping Jess to tidy the bedroom. He was busy pulling items out of the drawers as quickly as Jess was putting them away. Jess lifted Jason onto the bed so that she could put the last things away in the bathroom. Jason began jumping up and down on his parents' bed, getting more and more excited, when he fell backwards and hit his head on the bed head.

Jess ran into the bedroom when she heard his cry and comforted him straight away. Jason did not appear to have any sign of injury but was very upset and needed a lot of comforting before he would stop crying. Jess took him downstairs and gave him a treat and a drink of milk. Jason appeared to have recovered but as the morning wore on he became more irritable. He kept wanting to lie down but then would become restless and cry. Jess was getting somewhat concerned as this was not Jason's normal behaviour.

Jess decided to make an appointment with the GP. An appointment was made within the hour and Jason was seen straight away.

The GP found that Jason was indeed irritable but had no obvious sign of injury. Jason was uninterested in what the GP was doing and at times sat quietly on Jess's lap.

The GP was not happy with the way Jason was behaving and decided that he should go to hospital for observations.

Jess rang Ian straight away and they took Jason to hospital for 24-h observation. When Jason got to the ward he perked up when he saw all the toys.

Question one: Identify the coma scales that can be used with children across the age range.

5 minutes

Question two: Describe the neurological assessment one would make on Jason.

20 minutes

Time Allocation: **25 minutes**

Answer to question one:
Identify the coma scales that can be used with children across the age range.

The signs and symptoms of head injury stem from the insidious development of cerebral oedema. As Jason's cranium will not yet be fully formed and may still be pliable, rising intracranial pressure (ICP) can go relatively unnoticed for 6–18 h (Patterson *et al.*, 1992). It is for this reason that the nurse should regularly assess Jason's neurological status.

One of the most commonly used neurological assessment tools is the Glasgow Coma Scale (GCS) devised by Teasdale & Jennett (1974), which identifies three categories for assessment:

- Eye opening
- Best verbal response
- Best motor response

However, it became rapidly apparent that children and infants did not respond verbally or physically in the same way as adults because of their developmental immaturity. With this in mind, various modifications have been made to the GCS.

The neurological tools most commonly used with children and infants are the modified Pinderfield scale (Ferguson-Clark & Williams, 1998), the Adelaide scale (Williams, 1992) and the James scale (Patterson *et al.*, 1992) (Boxes 9.1–3).

Box 9.1. Adelaide scale.

Eyes open:
- Spontaneously: 4
- To speech: 3
- To pain: 2
- None: 1

Best verbal responses:
- Orientated: 5
- Words: 4
- Vocal sounds: 3
- Cries: 2
- None: 1

Best motor response:
- Obeys commands: 5
- Localizes to pain: 4
- Flexion to pain: 3
- Extension to pain: 2
- None: 1

Box 9.2. Pinderfield scale.

Respiration:
4 Normal, spontaneous and regular
3 Hyperventilation or shallow but regular
2 Cheyne Stokes or variably irregular
1 Inadequate spontaneous ventilation requiring support
0 Ventilation requiring support

Alertness (a measure of rousability shown by facial flinching, respiratory or limb movement):
5 Fully alert, immediately responds
4 Drowsy but easily roused by speech or gentle shaking
3 Rousable by shout or firm shake
2 Unrousable by shout, rousable by superficial shake
1 No eye opening even to pain

Eyes:
5 Spontaneous eye opening and looking at people
4 Spontaneous eye opening but not looking at people
3 Opens eyes in response to normal speech or voices
2 Opens eyes to shout
1 Not looking at people and only opens eyes to pain

Behaviour:
4 Obeys appropriate commands
3 Immediate appropriate response to simple commands/stimulation
2 Delayed response to repeated simple commands/stimulation
1 Doubtful/inappropriate response to stimulation/simple commands
0 No obedience/behavioural responses

Orientation/responses:
4 Recognizes and responds normally to significant persons/objects, eyes follow moving objects
3 Memory loss/withdrawn and uncooperative/occasional fixed eye contact
2 Seems confused/irritable
1 Unresponsive to staff/significant persons or name
0 Too drowsy to assess

Speech:
5 Answers simple questions/says appropriate words/smiles/coos
4 Inappropriate words/refuses to talk/irritable cry
3 Inappropriate cries/screams
2 Screams (high pitched)
1 Incomprehensible sounds/grunts
0 No sounds

Best motor response (stronger side):
7 Brisk movement/full power/purposeful localizing/useful response. Normal flexion in baby
6 Impaired postural maintenance/some weakness/sluggish pain localization with withdrawal
5 Non-localizing withdrawal
4 Abnormal flexion with non-purposeful response to pain
3 Brisk extensor posturing with no withdrawal
2 Sluggish extensor posturing/no withdrawal
1 Only a flicker to pain
0 None

Poorer motor response (weaker side):
BMR – PMR = measure of severity of hemiparesis. Each section should be appropriate for children of 6 months to 10 years of age

Box 9.3. James scale.

Score	Infant (preverbal)	Child
Eye opening:		
4	opens eyes spontaneously	opens eyes spontaneously
3	opens eyes to speech	opens eyes to speech
2	opens eyes to pain	opens eyes to pain
1	no response	no response
= Score		
Motor responses:		
6	spontaneous movements	obeys commands
5	withdraws to touch	localizes (purposeful movement)
4	withdraws from pain	withdraws from pain
3	abnormal flexion	abnormal flexion
2	abnormal extension	abnormal extension
1	no response	no response
= Score		
Verbal responses:		
5	coos, babbles, or cries appropriately	oriented, appropriate use of words
4	irritable cry	confused
3	cries only to pain	inappropriate use of words
2	moans to pain	incomprehensive use of words
1	no response	no response
= Score		
= Total score		

As can be seen these tools are similar but each is more age specific than the original GCS.

When used serially, the scores obtained using one of the tools will highlight a trend of either improving or deteriorating consciousness.

Regardless of which tool is being used, the nurse needs to have experience and knowledge in the use of these to gain an accurate neurological assessment (Ferguson-Clarke & Williams, 1998).

Answer to question two:
Describe the neurological assessment one would make on Jason.

Assessing Jason can begin straight away, by watching him play and the way in which he interacts with his parents. Ferguson-Clarke & Williams (1998) stated that these observations were a reliable baseline. It is important to take a history, so that Jason's developmental stage is recorded. As with any emergency situation, Jason should be assessed using the airway, breathing and circulation (ABC) protocol. It is vital to ensure that the oxygen supply to the brain is maintained as demand is increased following injury.

As Jason is currently alert, talking and running around, it is apparent that he can maintain his airway adequately. However, on-going assessment of this is essential. At this stage a primary neurological assessment followed by a detailed examination should be undertaken.

The initial assessment should include level of consciousness, pupil size and reaction to light, response to stimulation and ability to open eyes and verbalize to command. A simple mnemonic such as 'AVPU' (Patterson et al., 1992) can prove invaluable in this process:

A alert: responds to parents, strangers and new environment appropriately
V responds to verbal stimulation, may be sleepy but rousable
P responds to painful stimuli but unresponsive to surroundings
U unresponsive: no voluntary response to external stimuli

Jason's stage of development must always be uppermost in the nurse's mind as this will affect both the findings and interpretation of results. At 18 months of age, Jason should have a vocabulary of 200–300 words, which he can use to demonstrate an awareness of his surroundings.

A more detailed examination of neurological function should then follow (Box 9.4).

Box 9.4. Cranial nerves.

Cranial nerve	Function	Manifestations of damage	Assessment
I Olfactory	smell	loss of sense of smell (anosmia)	use of familiar smelling material to test (e.g. chocolate)
II Optic	vision	loss of visual acuity and defects to the visual field.	pupil reaction and size (see below); ask child to identify common objects near and far; test each eye separately
III Oculomotor	movement of eyelid and eyeball; constriction of pupil	strabismus (squint); ptosis (drooping eyelid); pupil dilation; involuntary eyeball movement downwards and outwards; diplopia (double vision)	look at the child; awareness of any predisposing abnormality or visual aid; pen torch to test constriction; record measurement diagrammatically or in millimetres; make child track eyes around objects
IV Trochlear	movement of eyeball	head tilt to affected side; possible diplopia and strabismus	as for cranial nerve III
V Trigeminal	chewing and sensation of touch, pain and temperature	paralysis of chewing muscles; loss of sensation	with eyes covered apply sharp and soft objects to the child's face; observe during eating
VI Abducens	movement of eyeball	eye cannot move laterally and is usually directed laterally	make sure the child keeps head still then track eyes through visual field
VII Facial	facial expression, saliva and tear secretion	facial paralysis (Bell's palsy): loss of taste; eyes open even during sleep	make faces to assess symmetry; salt, vinegar to test taste
VIII Vestibulocochlear	hearing and balance	tinnitus; vertigo, ataxia, nystagmus	test hearing by clap; ticking watch
IX Glossopharnygeal	taste, BP regulation, tear secretion	pain on swallowing; loss of taste and sensation in throat	evaluate cough, gag and swallow; check clarity of speech
X Vagus	visceral muscle movement	loss of swallowing and vocal cord movement; inability to interpret sensation from body organs	as for cranial nerve IX
XI Accessory	swallowing and head movement	inability to turn head or raise shoulders	ask child to turn head and shrug
XII Hypoglossal	tongue movement during speech and swallowing	difficulty in swallowing, speech and chewing	ability to stick out tongue

When observing Jason's pupils, their size should be noted before applying a light stimulus. The expected size of pupils throughout childhood is 2–4 mm at rest (Hazinski, 1999), and they would usually be equal unless the child has a predisposing ophthalmic problem. However, unequal pupils with an altered mental status can also indicate a space-occupying lesion such as a haematoma (Hazinski, 1999).

A child's natural curiosity will often lead them to open their eyes when a nurse approaches. On the other hand, after they have been examined a number of times, they may decide to keep their eyes tightly closed.

Motor response

It is important to observe the way in which Jason is sitting, and whether he is using his limbs spontaneously and symmetrically (Wong *et al.*, 1999). In addition, abnormal posture should be reported as primitive postural reflexes emerge as control over motor function is lost. The abnormality results when strong muscles overcome weak muscles. With decorticate posturing (Figure 9.1, left), the limbs are drawn into the midline and indicate cerebral cortex damage. Decerebrate posturing (Figure 9.1, right) is a sign of midbrain damage and is characterized by limbs being extended outwards from the body. It is important to be aware of responses that are normal in infancy, but abnormal in adults (Lower, 1992) such as Babinski's reflex in which the infant's toes hyperextend and fan out when the sole of the foot is stroked from heel to toe. This reflex is an abnormal finding after 1 year of age (Wong *et al.*, 1999).

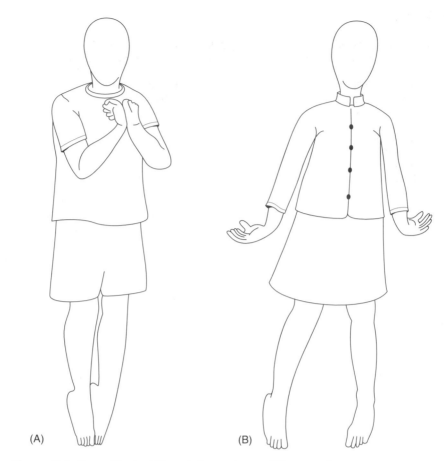

Figure 9.1. Decorticate (A) and decerebrate (B) posturing.

Vital signs

In addition to the above observations, the nurse will monitor Jason's vital signs. His pulse, respirations and BP should be recorded at intervals dictated by his current condition although custom and practice recommends at least hourly initially. A trend of falling pulse rate and increasing BP, accompanied by a decreasing level of consciousness can be indicative of rising ICP. This pattern, however, is not always apparent with children (Hazinski, 1999). Slow shallow respirations are associated with brain stem injury (Patterson *et al.*, 1992).

With regard to BP, Courts (1996), in her literature review, highlighted the unreliability of children's BP monitoring by indirect means and reminded nurses to ignore cuff sizes. She advocated opting for one cuff individual to the child, containing a bladder, which would cover the circumference of the limb used.

References

Courts, S. (1996). Monitoring blood pressure in children. *Paediatric Nursing*, 8, 25–27.

Ferguson-Clark, L., & Williams, C. (1998). Neurological assessment in children. *Paediatric Nursing*, 10, 29–35.

Hazinski, M. F. (1999). *Nursing Care of the Critically Ill Child*. London: Mosby.

Lower, J. S. (1992). Rapid neuro assessment. *American Journal of Nursing*, 92, 38–45.

Patterson, R. J., Brown, G. W., Salassi-Scotter, M., & Middaugh, D. (1992). Head injury in the conscious child. *American Journal of Nursing*, 92, 22–30.

Tatman, A., Warren, A., Williams, A., Powell, J. E., & Whithouse, W. (1997). Development of a modified Paediatric Coma Scale in intensive care: clinical practice. *Archives of Diseases in Childhood*, 77, 519–521.

Teasdale, G., & Jennett, B. (1974). Assessment of coma and impaired consciousness. *Lancet*, 2, 81–84.

Williams, J. (1992). Assessment of head injured children. *British Journal of Nursing*, 1, 82–84.

Wong, D. L., Hockenberry-Eaton, M., Wilson, D., Winkelstein, M. L., Ahmann, E., & DiVito-Thomas, P. A. (1999). *Whaley & Wong's Nursing Care of Infants and Children*, 6th edn. St Louis: Mosby.

Further reading

Harrison, M. (1991). The minor head injury. *Paediatric Nursing*, 3, 15–19.

Hofer, T. (1993). Glasgow Scale relationships in paediatric and adult patients. *Journal of Neuroscience Nursing*, 25, 218–227.

Martin, K. (1994). When the nurse says 'He's just not right': patient cues used by expert nurses to identify mild head injury. *Journal of Neuroscience Nursing*, 26, 210–217.

Trauma, sickle cell and postoperative observations of manipulated fracture

Jane McConochie

Selina Robiero is a 2-year-old African-Caribbean girl who has fallen off a climbing frame and injured her right arm. She has been admitted to the ward from A&E with a fracture of the mid-shaft of the radius and ulna of her right arm.

In A&E Selina was given Oramorph as an oral analgesic to relieve the pain. An X-ray was taken of the arm, which showed a simple fracture with a degree of displacement. It was explained to Mrs Robiero that Selina would need a manipulation under general anaesthetic (MUA) and consent was obtained for this. To help keep the arm comfortable a plaster of Paris backslab was applied and then the arm placed in a broad arm sling. As Selina is of African-Caribbean origin, blood was taken to check whether she had sickle cell anaemia, although when questioned her mother said that she had not shown any signs of the disease.

On admission to the ward Selina was quiet and very shy. She did not seem to be in any pain. Having admitted Selina to the ward, the nurse then prepared her for theatre. The result of the blood test was telephoned through to the ward and was negative.

On return to the ward Selina had her right arm in a full above-elbow plaster. The theatre staff also noted that Selina had head lice. Selina recovered from the anaesthetic and her arm was elevated in a Bradford sling and she was monitored to ensure that should complications occur they were quickly detected.

Question one: Why is it important that Selina's sickle cell status is known?

15 minutes

Question two: Describe the postoperative observations Selina would require to ensure early detection of complications.

20 minutes

Question three: Outline current principles of treatment for head lice (*Pediculus humanus capitis*).

25 minutes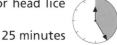

Time Allocation: **1 hour**

Answers to question one:
Why is it important that Selina's sickle cell status is known?

Although Selina's mother says that Selina has not displayed any signs of the disease in the past, this does not indicate what her sickle cell status is. For the first 6–12 months of life, Selina would still have fetal haemoglobin within her circulation and this would protect her red blood cells from sickling (Mayfield, 1999). Selina may have sickle cell trait rather than sickle cell disease. If Selina has either sickle cell disease or sickle cell trait, then she is at risk during an anaesthetic as any action that reduces oxygenation of the blood is likely to cause sickling (Wong *et al.*, 1999).

If Selina has sickle cell disease, then dehydration can cause her to produce sickle cells by raising the concentration of haemoglobin S within the red blood cells (Olujohungbe *et al.*, 1999). The risk of sickling is also increased with infection and by the demands placed on the body by wound healing (Wong *et al.*, 1999). It is, therefore, imperative that Selina's sickle cell status is known before any anaesthetic is delivered and to ensure that she remains hydrated. See also Profile 24 (Gemma Daniels).

Answer to question two:
Describe the postoperative observations Selina would require to ensure early detection of complications.

It is important postoperatively to monitor Selina's circulation and sensation to ensure that there is no impairment to either of these systems. To help this process McRae (1994) offered a classification that he called the five 'P's':

- Pain: following manipulation the patient is usually almost pain-free. If pain persists, this indicates a possible problem particularly if analgesics are not effective
- Paralysis: if finger movements are difficult, painful or absent, this indicates a problem
- Paraesthesia: loss of sensation in the fingers indicates nerve impairment
- Pallor: indicates impaired circulation
- Perishing cold: indicates circulatory impairment

Often all that is needed to relieve these symptoms is to split the plaster cast, which in turn relieves the pressure, circulation then immediately returning. If this does not occur, then surgical intervention will almost certainly be necessary. Immediate action is necessary as failure to do so could impair healing and may cause permanent damage.

Answer to question three:
Outline current principles of treatment for head lice
(*Pediculus humanus capitis*).

The head louse is a small parasite that lives on human heads. The louse feeds on blood ~4 hourly by biting capillaries on the scalp. The lice are ~0.5 cm in length and have six clawed legs that enable them to grasp the shafts of the hair and hold on. They survive for ~30 days laying their eggs (nits) at about 10 per day at the hair shaft where they become tightly adherent. After 1 week the nits hatch and nymphs emerge. The nymph is a smaller replica of the adult and takes another week to mature to adult form (PHLS, 1999).

It is rare, although not unheard of, for children of African-Caribbean families to have head lice. It is thought that the structure of their hair prevents the louse from holding on.

Girls appear to be more likely to have head lice than boys as they are more likely to have close contact with each other and share personal possessions (Anon., n.d.). The main symptom is itching, which may not present for up to 3 months (Aston *et al.*, 1998).

Treatments should be preventative and corrective (Carter & Dearmun, 1995).

- Preventative: brush and comb the child's hair thoroughly at least twice a day and wash regularly with normal shampoo. Check everyone in the family at least once a week. Use a fine toothed detector comb. Using conditioner may make this easier
- Corrective: if live lice are found, then treatment should be carried out. There are two possible forms of treatment (given below)

Conditioner method

The hair is washed as normal and then hair conditioner is liberally applied. The hair is divided into a small section and a comb with very fine teeth (known as a nit comb) is used to comb the hair from the roots, covering small areas at a time. When all of the head has been covered the hair can be rinsed and dried as normal. This treatment needs to be repeated every third day for 2 weeks (Livingstone, n.d.).

Chemical method

This uses special lotions (e.g. Derbac-M, Prioderm) to kill the adult louse and prevent re-infection. These lotions contain Malathion, which is an organophosphate about which health concerns have been raised, for in the laboratory when used on rats it has been found to be carcinogenic. These chemicals should only be used if live lice are seen. They should be used in accordance with the manufacturer's instructions and should not be used repeatedly (Cook, 1998).

References

Anon. (n.d., accessed 25 July 2000). Lice
[http://onhealth.com/conditions/resource/conditions/item,395.as].
Aston, R., Duggal, H., & Simpson, J. (1999, accessed 26 July 2000). Head lice: a report for
consultants in communicable disease control (CCDCs) [http://www.fam-
english.demon.co.uk/phmeghl.htm].
Carter, B., & Dearmun, A. K. (eds) (1995). *Child Health Care Nursing*. Oxford: Blackwells.
Cook, R. (1998). Treatment of head lice. *Paediatric Nursing*, 10, 29–33.
Livingstone, R. (n.d., accessed 25 July 2000). Head lice and nits
[http://web.ukonline.co.uk/ruth.livingstone/little/headlice.htm].
Mayfield, E. (1999, accessed 26 July 2000). New hope for people with sickle cell anemia
[http://www.fda.gov/fdac/features/496_sick.htm].
McRae, R. (1994, accessed 26 July 2000). *Practical Fracture Treatment*, 3rd edn. London:
Churchill Livingstone.
Olujohungbe, A., Yardumian, A., & Cinkotai, K. I. (1999, accessed 26 July 2000). New
treatment strategies for sickle cell disease
[http://www.sicklecellsociety.org/resnrep.htm].
Public Health Laboratory Service (1999, accessed 26 July 2000). 'Wired for Health' head lice
(pediculosis) [http://www.phls.co.uk/advice/wfhheadlice.htm].
Wong, D., Hockenberry-Eaton, M., Wilson, D., Winkelstein, M. L., Ahmann, E., & DiVito-
Thomas, P. (1999). *Whaley and Wong's Nursing Care of Infants and Children*, 6th edn. St
Louis: Mosby.

Further reading

Sowen, P. (1999). Head lice: new developments on a controversial issue. *Professional Care of
Mother and Child*, 9, 146–148.

Manipulated fracture

Fussy eating behaviour and food refusal

Leigh F. Caws

Patrick Cooper is 3 years old and the second child in the family. He has an older brother, Craig, aged 7, and his mother had a baby girl, Anna, 10 weeks ago. Patrick was weaned traditionally within the recommendations of the DoH Report (1994), but always demonstrated a clear preference towards the sweeter foods that his mother tried to discourage. His mother has very well formed ideas about sweets and confectionery in her childrens' diet, which they are allowed infrequently as a special treat. Since ~15 months of age, Patrick has been fussy with his food and is demonstrating an increasing reluctance to explore new foods and eat what his parents would consider an adequate diet. This is causing great concern to them, resulting in confrontations at mealtimes and temper tantrums at the table. His mother finds that she is spending half the day chasing him around, coaxing him with a variety of tempting healthy foods which she has invariably taken great pains to prepare. Patrick is cared for predominantly by his mother as his father is a long-distance lorry driver. The pressure of the new baby and Patrick's refusal of foods combined with her concern of his 'skinny' appearance is becoming unbearable for his mother, so she has arranged to see her health visitor. Patrick was weighed at the clinic at the same time as the baby. He was 12 kg, which was unchanged since the last measurement 6 months before and his height had increased from 91 to 93 cm during this time.

The health visitor asked Patrick's mother to provide a typical day's food diary on him (Table 11.1).

Table 11.1. Typical food diary for Patrick.

Time (hours)	Food	Weight/amount
07.00	Rice Krispies	15 g
	full cream milk	100 ml
	orange squash	200 ml
10.00	apple	half
	blackcurrant juice (no added sugar)	200 ml
12.00	peanut butter sandwich (white bread)	30 g (bread); 10 g (peanut butter)
	Flora Light spread	5 g
	yoghurt (Ski – low fat)	half pot
	orange squash	200 ml
15.00	apple	quarter
	blackcurrant juice	200 ml
17.30	baked beans	30 g
	chicken nuggets	one nugget
	banana	quarter
	orange squash	200 ml
19.00	orange squash	200 ml
	cheddar cheese	28 g

Question one: Discuss the significance of Patrick's weight in relation to his age.

10 minutes

Question two: Calculate the calorific value and the protein, fat and carbohydrate content of Patrick's diet.

20 minutes

Question three: Make a judgement on the nutritional adequacy of Patrick's diet using the COMA Report on Nutritional Guidelines (DoH, 1991).

10 minutes

Question four: Parents are responsible for what their children are offered to eat, how much they are offered to eat and how they promote eating behaviour, but the child decides how much to eat, whether to eat what is put in front of them and controls his/her behavioural responses. Rationalize the advice and guidance one might offer to the family to overcome Patrick's eating problems, which is considerate of these issues.

30 minutes

Time Allowance: **1 hour 10 minutes**

Answer to question one:
Discuss the significance of Patrick's weight in relation to his age.

By plotting Patrick's weight and height on a child growth foundation chart (1996) for boys it can be established that he is on the 25th centile for his height and between the 0.4th and 2nd centile for his weight. The increase in height and the static weight for the past 6 months might give rise to Patrick's slightly emaciated appearance and in one sense this might be reassuring to the parents as linear growth has occurred appropriately. Linear growth is considered one of the reliable measurements of general growth and by 3 years of age this should be fairly stable (Campbell & Glasper, 1995). Weight and height should be relative; therefore, it would be ideal if Patrick's weight was nearer to 14 kg. His weight should give cause for concern and be monitored on a monthly basis.

Answer to question two:
Calculate the calorific value and the protein, fat and carbohydrate content of Patrick's diet.

Table 11.2 shows the approximate energy value and quantities of protein, fat and carbohydrate calculated for Patrick's diet based on his food diary.

Table 11.2. Dietary analysis.

Food	Quantity	kcal	Protein (g)	Fat (g)	Carbohydrate (g)
Rice Krispies	15 g	57.3	0.9	0.105	13.2
Full-cream milk	100 ml	66	3.3	3.8	4.7
Orange squash	800 ml	44	0.08	0	9.6
Apple	half	40	0	0.5	10
Blackcurrant juice (no added sugar)	400 ml	6	0.15	0	0.75
White bread	30 g	80	2.5	1.2	15
Peanut butter	10 g	61	2.78	5	1.2
Margarine spread (light)	5 g	18	0.005	1.9	0.18
Baked beans	30 g	30	2	0.1	3.3
Chicken nuggets	one nugget	51	2.6	2.4	4.7
Banana	half	50	0.5	0	13
Cheddar cheese	28 g	115	7	9	0
Yoghurt (low fat)	about half a pot	55	2.5	0.75	10
Totals		673.3	24.315	24.76	85.63

Answer to question three:

Make a judgement on the nutritional adequacy of Patrick's diet using the COMA Report on Nutritional Guidelines (DoH, 1991).

Patrick is consuming only half the estimated average requirements of calories for his age and sex, which would account for his failure to gain weight. His protein consumption is twice the requirement. He is, however, eating adequate amounts of carbohydrate and fat, but the carbohydrate and fat content of the diet could be increased to boost calorie intake encouraging weight gain, particularly if he is a very active. Table 11.3 shows the comparison between the recommended estimated average requirements for a child of Patrick's age and Patrick's actual energy, protein, fat and carbohydrate intake.

Table 11.3. Analysis of Patrick's actual intake.

Nutrient	Estimated average requirements (EAR)	Actual intake
kcal	1230 kcal day^{-1}	673.3 kcal day^{-1}
Protein	11.7 g day^{-1}	24.3 g day^{-1}
Fat	constitutes 22% of energy intake per day	24.8 g day^{-1} (22.4% of energy intake)
Carbohydrate	50–100 g day^{-1}	85.6 g day^{-1}

Answer to question four:

Parents are responsible for what their children are offered to eat, how much they are offered to eat and how they promote eating behaviour, but the child decides how much to eat, whether to eat what is put in front of them and controls his/her behavioural responses. Rationalize the advice and guidance one might offer the family to overcome Patrick's eating problem, which is considerate of these issues.

What Patrick should be offered, based on the assessment of his dietary intake, to ensure adequate weight gain proportional to his height is more fatty and carbohydrate foods. Nutritious high-fat foods should not be limited in this age group provided saturated fats from foods such as chocolate, crisps, cakes and chips are kept to a minimum (Thompson, 1998). Fatty foods that should be encouraged in the diet include full-cream milk, yoghurt, cheese, meat, small amounts of butter and vegetable oils. These foods are also rich in calcium along with baked beans, pulses, peanut butter, *fromage frais*, peas, broccoli and white bread to help build strong bones and teeth. Avoid preparatory diet foods such as low fat yoghurt and spreads. The *National Diet and Nutritional Survey: Children Aged 1½–4½* (MAFF, 1995) identified low iron intakes as a problem in this age group, especially in the form of haem iron found in red meat and offal, which are two foods that preschool children and toddlers dislike due to difficulty in chewing. Patrick might well be at risk of developing anaemia, so other more palatable foods to this age group such as minced meat (in various forms), roast chicken, Weetabix, white bread, broccoli and the occasional treat of dark chocolate might be appealing. When increasing the carbohydrate component of the diet, non-milk extrinsic sugars such as sweets, cakes, fizzy drinks and biscuits should be kept to a minimum to avoid dental caries and should never be used as a reward for good behaviour or as a bribe (Thompson, 1998).

How much to eat: toddlers and preschool children require less energy per kg body weight than infants; therefore, it is perfectly reasonable to expect a reduction in appetite. At 3 years of age, children are easily put off by certain smells, tastes, unappealing appearances and large portions. It is unreasonable for Patrick to eat three square meals a day; small snacks and meals are more appealing. Desserts should not be withheld under the threat of not finishing the main course.

How to promote good eating behaviour and control responses: initially, one must ascertain who has the problem of refusing food, as invariably it is the parent who is anxious and concerned and not the child. Skilful discussion should take place with the parents so that they can deduce this for themselves and take ownership of the issues. Guidance to the parents might take the following forms:

- Make mealtimes a family social occasion at the table with discussion on the days events thus avoiding confrontation with Patrick and taking the pressure off eating

- Prepare simple meals to avoid the frustration experienced by the parents
- If the child refuses food, just take the plate away. Do not force the child to eat and do not chase around after it offering alternatives
- Reward good behaviour with an exciting activity and ignore undesirable behaviour
- Allow the child to eat with its peers who eat well, but do not pressurize them to follow their behaviour
- Provide vitamin supplements to be taken with food
- Engage the child in cooking and food preparation activities such as making his own sandwiches, cake making and putting the toppings on their own pizza
- Avoid asking the child to eat when they are engrossed in play activities, which they would rather be doing
- Discreetly record the child's food intake occasionally to provide reassurance
- Record height and weight monthly
- Reassure parents that the problem will resolve naturally if it is not made into a battleground

References

Campbell, S., & Glasper, E. A. (1995). *Whaley and Wong's Children's Nursing*. London: Mosby.

Child Growth Foundation (1996). *Boys Four-in-One Growth Charts*. London: CGF.

Department of Health (1991). *Dietary Reference Values for Food Energy and Nutrients for the United Kingdom*. Report on Health and Social Subjects no. 41. London: HMSO.

Department of Health (1994). *Weaning and Weaning Diet*. Report on Health and Social Subjects no. 45. Committee on Medical Aspects of Food Policy. London: HMSO.

Ministry of Agriculture, Fisheries and Food (MAFF) (1995). *National Diet and Nutritional Survey: Children Aged 1½–4½*, vol. 1. London: HMSO.

Thompson, P. (1998). *Nutritional Requirements of Infants and Young Children: Practical Guidelines*. Oxford: Blackwells.

Further reading

Daws, D. (1994). Family relationships and infant feeding problems. *Health Visitor*, 67, 162–164.

Douglas, J. E. and Bryan, M. (1996). Interview data on severe behavioural eating difficulties in young children. *Archives of Disease in Childhood*, 75, 304–308.

Glod, C. A. (1993). Long term consequences of childhood physical and sexual abuse. *Archives of the Psychiatric Nurse*, 7, 163–173.

Lask, B. and Bryant-Waugh, R. (1995). A European perspective on eating disorders. *Journal of Adolescent Health*, 16, 418–419.

McCann, H. (1994). Eating habits and attitudes of mothers of children with non-organic failure to thrive. *Archives of Disease in Childhood*, 70, 234–236.

Satter, E. (1995). Feeding dynamics: helping children to eat. *Journal of Pediatric Health Care*, 9, 178–184.

Southall, A., & Schwartz, A. (2000). *Feeding Problems in Children*. London: Radcliffe Medical.

Three-year-old with diabetes

Ruth Sadik

Gareth Jones is 3 years old and lives at home with his parents, Karen and Mark. He has a brother, Godfrey, aged 11 years. Despite the age difference, the boys are very close and Karen has noticed that Godfrey often gives Gareth some of his sweets and crisps as Gareth is constantly hungry. He also has an enormous appetite at mealtimes. Godfrey has been becoming impatient with Gareth recently, as he only wants to sit around and says he is too tired to play football. His parents have also noticed that he has become less energetic over the past 4 weeks and is extremely thirsty and is always going to the toilet.

During the past 3 weeks, Gareth, who is normally potty trained, has been having wet beds every night and Karen is getting to the end of her tether with her youngest son. Wendy, the health visitor, explains to Karen that the more cross she gets with Gareth, the more likely he is to continue wetting.

This morning, Gareth awoke with abdominal pain and vomited copiously. His mother noticed that he appeared drowsy, and when she went to comfort him noted that he had smelly breath. Adding up all the factors that had been affecting her son over the past month, Karen decided to take Gareth to the GP.

While at the surgery, Gareth requests to use the toilet and the doctor asked that the practice nurse test the urine sample. It was quickly established that Gareth had glucose and ketones in his urine. The GP undertook a blood test, which revealed a blood glucose level of 25 mmol litre^{-1}, and he informed Gareth and his mother that he suspected diabetes and immediately referred them to the local hospital.

On admission to the ward, it is ascertained by further blood tests that Gareth has C-reactive protein, indicating insulin-dependent diabetes. His electrolytes are imbalanced with a potassium of 6.8 mmol litre^{-1} (normal 3.5–5.5 mmol litre^{-1}) (Evans, 1994).

Question one: Explain the pathophysiology of insulin-dependent diabetes mellitus (IDDM).

15 minutes

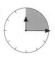

Question two: Outline diabetic keto-acidosis (DKA).

10 minutes

Question three: Describe the potential long-term complications of IDDM.

15 minutes

Question four: Describe the information that Gareth and his family will require to manage his condition safely at home.

1 hour

Time Allowance: **1 hour 40 minutes**

Answer to question one:
Explain the pathophysiology of insulin-dependent diabetes mellitus (IDDM).

IDDM or Type 1 diabetes is the most common endocrine disorder in children with an incidence rate of 1:2500 aged < 5 years, increasing to 1:300 by 18 years of age (Faulkner & Clark, 1998). About three-quarters of all newly diagnosed cases of diabetes occur in children < 18 years of age, and according to Challener (1998a, b) the incidence in the UK is increasing rapidly, and occurring more predominantly in younger children (McEvilley, 1997). Management of the condition needs to be integrated with the physical and emotional needs of children, adolescents and their families.

In health, insulin is produced by specialized endocrine cells of the pancreas, known as β-cells. It is composed of two peptide chains, A and B, which are connected by a disulphide bond, the C or connecting peptide (Kapit *et al.*, 1998). When insulin is released from the β-cells of the pancreas it is bound to β-globulin, which enables it to facilitate the entry of glucose into the cells, maintaining normal fasting blood glucose levels of 2.5–5.6 mmol litre^{-1} (Evans, 1994). However, being bound to a protein also makes it inactive if administered via the mouth (Harrop *et al.*, 1999).

Insulin is released in response to the level of glucose in the blood. As the level of glucose in the blood rises, following a meal or snack, the β-cells of the pancreas detect this and release insulin to facilitate the uptake of glucose by the tissues. This action results in reduced blood glucose levels. While many tissues such as the brain, renal tubules and intestinal mucosa can utilize glucose without insulin being present, if it is absent, muscle and adipose tissues are impermeable to glucose.

Diabetes is a syndrome of relative or absolute insulin deficiency and is hallmarked by persistent hyperglycaemia. The treatment is aimed at lowering blood glucose levels to normal or near normal levels through a complex regimen of insulin injections, blood glucose monitoring, a carbohydrate restricted healthy diet and exercise (Lowes & Lyne, 1999).

While the cause of IDDM is relatively unknown, what is known is that it is a multifactoral autoimmune disorder, resulting in pancreatic islet cell inability to produce insulin. When 90% of the β-cells are affected, IDDM becomes noticeable. This variety is also frequently associated with specific human leukocyte antigen (HLA) types with a predisposition to viral insulitis or autoimmune (islet cell antibody) phenomenon and leaves the child prone to ketosis.

One theory (Yki-Jarvinen, 1994) explains causation as occurring once the β-cells are damaged, as at this time they release an auto-antigen recognized as non-self. This, along with the specific HLA molecules, is presented to the macrophages, resulting in the release of various lymphokinins. This reaction causes T- and B-lymphocytes to produce antibodies against the β-cells, which decreases the amount of insulin produced. However, others (Cradock, 1995; Challener, 1998a) identified that a resistance to insulin might be the main cause.

The effects of decreased insulin secretion are:

- Incomplete oxidation of glucose
- Hyperglycaemia

- Glycosuria when blood sugar levels > 11 mmol l^{-1}
- Diuresis is initiated, which might lead to dehydration
- Protein and fat are oxidized
- Ketones accumulate in the blood
- Ketonuria is evident

The effects of depleted insulin can be explained by the fact that glucose entry into muscle and fat cells requires interplay between potassium and insulin. If insulin is deficient then potassium leaks out of the cell causing blood levels to rise, as sodium moves into the cell. As glucose cannot move into the cell hyperglycaemia occurs. This creates a negative intercellular gradient causing fluid to move from the cells to the interstitial space and then into the extracellular (glomerular) space, which is referred to as an osmotic diuresis. This in turn leads to classical signs and symptoms of IDDM of dehydration, polyuria, polydipsia and serum sodium depletion. Since glucose cannot enter the cell, fat is used as an alternative form of glucose in a process known as gluconeogenesis and it contributes to further hyperglycaemia. Cellular depletion of sugar is detected and the hunger mechanism is triggered adding further to the rising blood glucose levels.

Shortly after diagnosis, a honeymoon period of weeks or months is experienced by children with diabetes, where insulin secretion re-occurs, glucose and ketone uria disappear and the disease goes into remission. The duration of this phase increases with the age at onset of the disorder (Wiklund & Persson, 1999, citing Wallenstein *et al.*). Following this period of remission, the secretion of natural insulin once again decreases with a concomitant rise in the amount of injected insulin required.

Answer to question two:
Outline diabetic keto-acidosis (DKA).

DKA is a relatively common presenting feature of insulin-dependent diabetes. Despite recent advances in the management of IDDM, the incidence rate of DKA has not declined (Lebovitz, 1995).

As fat is converted to glucose, glycerol is transformed into ketone bodies, principally acetone, by the liver. The excess is excreted via the lungs and urinary system. As ketone bodies are acid radicals, their excess results in lowering the blood pH, leaving hydrogen ions free in the blood. These combine with bicarbonate to form carbonic acid, which when mixed with water forms carbon dioxide. The respiratory system attempts to eliminate excessive amounts of carbon dioxide by increasing the respiratory rate and depth, referred to as Kussmaul's respirations. The excreted acetone causes a new mown hay or fruity smell to be detected on the breath (Cradock, 1995; McEvilley, 1997; Harrop et al., 1999).

The kidneys compensate for the increased renal blood pH by increasing hydrogen production, causing blood pH to fall even further.

The kidney creating decreased blood levels excretes potassium, even though serum levels appear high due to resulting hypovolaemia. Low potassium might result in cardiac arrhythmias. The effects of acidosis are given in Figure 12.1.

The manifestations of both hyper- and hypoglycaemia are given in Box 12.1. Whatever the cause, correction of fluid and electrolyte balance requires immediate treatment.

Box 12.1. Manifestations of hypo- and hyperglycaemia.

DKA manifestation (hyperglycaemia)	**Diabetic coma (hypoglycaemia)**
Polydipsia	Hyperpnoea
Polyphagia and weight loss	Soft sunken eyeballs
Polyuria	Rigid abdomen
Recurrent *Candida*	Weak rapid pulse
Fatigue	Decreased temperature
Dry skin	Decreased BP
Skin and urinary infections	Abdominal pain

Management of diabetic keto-acidosis

The outcomes of treatment are to stabilize Gareth's condition by achieving metabolic control, rehydration and restoration of electrolyte balance.

Initial management

Gareth's initial management will depend on whether he is in shock or unconscious. If this is the case, the staff should initiate:

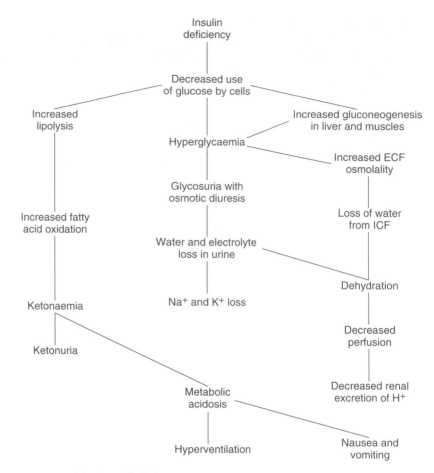

Figure 12.1. Acidosis and diabetes.

- Airway, breathing and circulation (ABC) first-aid (see Profile 25, Caroline Davis) and correct hypovolaemia with 10 ml kg⁻¹ colloid solution
- Observation of vital signs to include appearance, TPR, BP and neurological assessment
- IVI of isotonic saline, if Gareth is assessed as being >10% dehydrated and clinically acidotic. Calculations of his fluid requirements can be estimated using the formula in Profile 25 (Caroline Davies)
- Observation of urinary output as Gareth might require 0.9% sodium chloride to which 20 mmol potassium chloride is added to every 500 ml; if he is voiding, > 25 ml h⁻¹
- Oxygen via a face mask to help to reverse lactic acidosis
- Continuous IV insulin given on a sliding scale dependent on blood glucose level. It is normally calculated on 0.1 unit kg⁻¹ h⁻¹ for children aged ≥ 8 years, but as Gareth is only 3 years of age he will be administered 0.05 unit kg⁻¹ h⁻¹ (Harrop *et al.*, 1999). Although scales might vary depending on the paediatric specialist teams, Cradock (1995) identified that two factors must be taken into consideration:

- whole team understand the scale being used
- that there is no '0' on the scale (where insulin is turned off if the blood glucose level falls below a certain level) as she cautions that this can rapidly result in hyperglycaemia
- Nasogastric tube if required to decompress the stomach and reduce the risk of aspiration
- Hourly monitoring of Gareth's blood glucose levels
- Testing all urine for glucose and ketones
- Monitoring of renal output, which should be 1–2 ml kg^{-1} day^{-1}
- Assessment of neurological status (see Profile 9, Jason King) hourly to ensure that cerebral oedema is not developing
- Weighing twice daily to estimate degree of rehydration
- Recording of his ECG to observe for T-waves, which might show a widening of the QT interval or a flattened T-wave as a result of potassium imbalance
- Mouth care while Gareth is nil by mouth

The doctors would also assess electrolyte balance frequently during IV therapy.

Once blood pH and bicarbonate levels are within normal limits, sub-cutaneous insulin injections can be commenced.

Answer to question three:
Describe the potential long-term complications of IDDM.

Gareth's family will be advised about healthy eating, including a balance between carbohydrates that have the greatest effects on blood glucose level. HbA1c is used to evaluate blood glucose control over a protracted period. It is a reliable indicator of blood glucose levels over the preceding 2–3 months as red blood cells permeable to glucose convey it on Hb molecules for the life of that red cell. Given that these cells in health survive for ~120 days, testing Gareth for glycosylated Hb will estimate his degree of control and compliance (Selekman *et al.*, 1999). The higher HbA1c is, the poorer the glycaemic control over the period concerned. As the brain is still developing until 7 years of age, glycaemic control should be maximal to prevent hypoglycaemic episodes detrimental to brain growth. Control of blood glucose levels throughout childhood has been identified as the most important aspect in preventing long-term adverse effects (DCCTRG, 1994; Shield & Baum, 1998).

The long-term complications of diabetes can be separated into two groups, microvascular and macrovascular, a list of which is given in Box 12.2.

Box 12.2. Potential complications of IDDM.

Microvascular	**Macrovascular**
Retinopathy	Transient ischaemic attacks
Nephropathy	Strokes
Neuropathy:	Angina
	Myocardial infarction
	Intermittent claudication
	Ulceration
	Gangrene

Predisposing factors to the above are hypertension, obesity, smoking and hyperlipidaemia. It is, therefore, vital that Gareth avoids becoming overweight and is deterred from starting smoking. Health education with the whole family should be implemented.

Answer to question four:
Describe the information that Gareth and his family will require to manage his condition safely at home.

The onset of diabetes mellitus tends to occur unexpectedly, giving the family little time to adjust to the diagnosis, learn to respond to Gareth's illness and maintain family integrity over a relatively short period. The way in which they will respond to Gareth's condition depends on a variety of factors, such as:

- Their view of the world
- Family system and support
- Perception of the severity of diabetes
- Age and characteristics of affected child
- Extent of social and professional support

Children with diabetes and their families should receive treatment and care from a physician-coordinated team. The family will need to receive comprehensive training in self-management and intensive treatment programmes.

When teaching Gareth and his family the nurse must relinquish the caring role and become a facilitator employing listening and teaching skills (Cradock, 1995). Consideration must be given to the psycho-social determinants of health and illness (Brennan, 1996), and the nurse must recognize that stress interferes with the uptake and retention of information, necessitating repetition of facts and the presentation of information in written as well as verbal forms.

A plan should be devised with Karen and Mark to cover aspects such as:

- How to obtain and store insulin and insulin injection equipment
- How to draw up and administer insulin
- Use of asepsis
- Choice of injection sites
- Disposal of sharps
- Dietary aspects
- Sick day rules
- Dealing with hypoglycaemic episodes

Once the plan has been devised, Karen and Mark should be given instruction in manageable chunks with written information to back up both theory and practice.

Richmond (1998a) showed that parents experience distress, guilt and anxiety if their child's glucose levels are not maintained and feel that professionals equate poor control with poor compliance. They need staff to stop fixating on blood glucose levels and concentrate on the broader psychological aspects associated with instability and use more neutral language.

It has been shown by Hatton *et al.* (1995) that families containing a young child with diabetes often suffer social isolation as extended family members and friends are reluctant to baby-sit, in case the child becomes unwell. It has also been shown that parents of children with diabetes trust other adults less with their children and worry more (Gardner, 1998; Wiklund & Persson, 1999). This might be overcome by teaching the extended family about diabetes, injection techniques and hypoglycaemic episodes (Hatton *et al.*, 1995; Ingersoll & Golden, 1995).

Factors affecting glycaemic control are, therefore:

- Response to diagnosis
- Poor understanding of diabetes
- Family equilibrium
- Psychological problems
- Issues relating to puberty and adolescence

Support for Gareth and his family at home will include input from the multi-disciplinary team, which might involve:

- Children's community nurses
- Paediatric dietician
- Children's diabetic nurse
- Paediatrician
- Children's community psychiatric nurse
- GP
- School nurse and teacher

Children < 4 years of age lack the ability to recognize and respond to hypo-glycaemia (Weir *et al.*, 1994; Challener, 1998b) and intercurrent illness is more common, which increases the child's metabolic rate and, therefore, the need for carbohydrate. As much childhood illness results in unwillingness to eat or nausea and vomiting, sick-day management rules must be established. The principles of management for children who cannot take their full complement of carbohydrate are (Challener, 1998a; Richmond, 1999):

- Not to stop insulin
- Sugar-free drinks to prevent dehydration
- Blood glucose measurement before breakfast, lunch, tea and bed
- Urinary estimations of glucose and ketones
- Extra units of insulin if blood glucose level is high
- Liquid carbohydrate in cases of vomiting
- Contact GP in cases of:
    - vomiting for > 24 h
    - abdominal pain, drowsiness or breathing changes
    - blood glucose remains high and/or ketones persist in urine

Dietary guidelines

Over-aggressive dietary manipulation must be avoided in the young to prevent possible non-compliance in later teenage years (Weir *et al.*, 1994). The strategy currently advocated is to give small amounts of starchy food which the child wants at regular intervals (Richmond, 1998a).

The benefits of a paediatric dietician are:

- Meet Gareth's nutritional requirements for normal growth
- Optimize blood glucose level
- Devise individualized eating plan
- Educate family re healthy eating

Gareth's family is well advised about healthy eating, which will include a balance between carbohydrates, which have the greatest effects on blood glucose level, and fibre, which slows the absorption of glucose, fats and protein. Table 12.1 shows the recommendations regarding diet.

Table 12.1. Recommendations for diet.

Classification	Food stuff	Recommended amounts
Carbohydrate	bread, pasta, potatoes	40–45% energy requirements
	sugar	25 g day^{-1}
Fibre	fruit, peas, baked beans, cereals	2 g 100 kcal^{-1} day^{-1}
Fat	dairy produce, red meat, oils	30–35% energy requirements
Protein	pulses, meat, fish, eggs	13% of energy

As carbohydrates have the greatest impact on blood glucose levels, it is important to calculate the amount required on an age basis and spread the amount evenly across the day.

An approximate formula for carbohydrate requirements is:

120 g day^{-1} + 10 g for every year of age.

As Gareth is 3 years old he will need:

120 + 30 g = 150 g day^{-1}.

This would be spread across the day:

- Breakfast: 30 g
- Snack: 20 g
- Lunch: 30 g
- Snack: 20 g
- Tea: 30 g
- Snack: 20 g

There are two main approaches to diet (Richmond, 1998a):

- Qualitative: involves advocating a healthy eating plan based on three meals and three snacks per day. The diet should be geared to what the child and family normally eat with an emphasis on low-fat and high-fibre foods
- Quantitative carbohydrate exchanges: this is where the family is encouraged to recognize 10 g portions of carbohydrate, which can be exchanged for what the child prefers spread across three meals and three snacks. The method is best for families where average body weight does not fall within normal limits

Treatment of hypoglycaemia

This is difficult to detect in young children and its presentation is very individual. At Gareth's age, his day is relatively short and he is likely to experience spontaneous periods of high activity followed by sleep. This will make blood glucose control difficult, and the potential for hypoglycaemic episodes increases.

Hypoglycaemia presents as:

- Shaky
- Weakness
- Headache
- Hungry
- Sweaty
- Confused
- Blurred vision
- Irritable
- Vocal repetition
- Photophobia
- Lips and mouth might feel numb
- Abdominal pain

If conscious give glucose containing food: > 5 years of age, three glucose tablets; < 5 years of age, two or 60 ml Lucozade as 30 ml = 10 g carbohydrate. If the child refuses or cannot cooperate, squeeze Hypostop (40% glucose gel) into the cheek and massage into the mucus membrane to aid absorption. If the child does not respond within 10 min or is unconscious, give glucagon (a naturally occurring substance that helps convert stored glycogen into glucose) intramuscularly or subcutaneously, which takes 5–15 min to be effective.

All activity should be suspended for at least 30 min following recovery.

Many parents find hypoglycaemic episodes distressing and as a result keep their children with blood glucose levels higher than is recommended in an attempt to prevent them (Richmond, 1996).

Children can freely attend parties as the extra treats compensate for the added excitement and activity.

Insulin injections

Insulin is available in rapid, short, intermediate or long-acting types. While the first two are clear, the other types should appear cloudy but not contain sediment (ADA, 1997) (Table 12.2):

Table 12.2. Insulin characteristics.

Type of insulin	Duration (h)	Peak (h)
Soluble/short-acting	0.5–6	2–4
Isophane/intermediate	2–14	4–8
Long-acting	4–48	varies

- Insulin should not be kept at room temperature for > 1 month
- As insulin settles it should be rolled between the palms to mix and should not be shaken
- Local irritation at the injection site can be as a result of using cold insulin
- Rotate injection areas to prevent lipoatrophy. Insulin is most rapidly absorbed from the abdomen, then thighs, then arms

- Subcutaneous injections can be administered through a layer of clothing if necessary
- During growth spurts insulin needs are increased dramatically and blood glucose will be more difficult to control

Equipment must be sterile, hands and skin should be socially clean. Insulin should be administered into one of the sites shown in Figure 12.2 at either 90° if the child has a sufficient layer of subcutaneous tissue, or at 45–90° into a fold of skin if the child is particularly lean (Cradock, 1995; ADA, 1997).

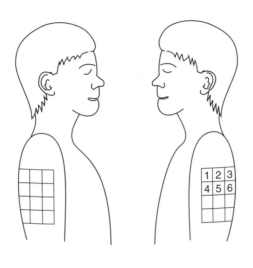

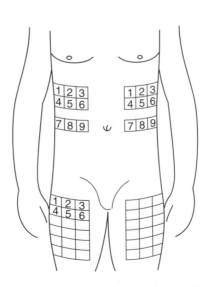

Figure 12.2. Subcutaneous insulin injection. Rotate through one area at a time.

Insulin absorption varies depending on the site of administration so when rotating sites this should be done around a single site (Figure 12.3) rather than, for example, the arm in the morning and thigh in the evening, which can result in unstable blood glucose levels. If the abdomen is used a 5-cm area around the naval should be avoided.

Disposal of sharps such as needles or lancets need to be disposed of in a puncture resistant disposable container.

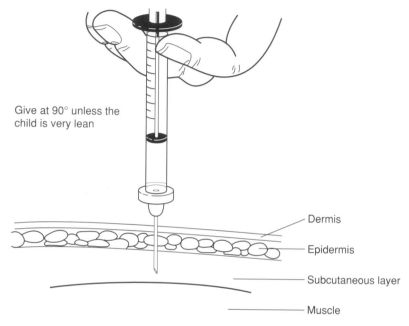

Give at 90° unless the child is very lean

Dermis

Epidermis

Subcutaneous layer

Muscle

Figure 12.3. Injection sites.

Exercise

The benefits of exercise are:

- Healthier cardiovascular system
- Improved blood glucose level control
- Increased insulin uptake
- Increased calcium uptake
- Decreased blood lipid levels
- Improved weight control

All normal sports are now possible and children now have national sporting heroes who are role models. Carbohydrate compensation is required before exercise to prevent hypoglycaemia. However, Challener (1998a, b) pointed out that school physical education sessions for young children are frequently cancelled at short notice and he cautions that the exercise of changing clothes and shoes does not equate to a Mars Bar!

Blood glucose monitoring

There is a variety of tools available to monitor blood glucose levels from a finger prick. Most are the preference of the child, family and should be taught according to the manufacturer's directions.

Day-to-day variations will depend on:

- Insulin absorption rate
- Exercise
- Stress
- Food absorption
- Hormonal change

As Gareth grows up, his parents need to be made aware of factors that he might experience as a result of being labelled as having diabetes. Miller (1999), in her study of children's views, identified these as:

- Dislike of daily discipline involving diet, injections and monitoring tests, which they identify as boring, time-consuming, eternal, responsible and imposing different restrictions on their lives
- Many children identified that absorption of the above factors into every day life by friends and family led them to feel a sense of sameness
- Good aspects of having diabetes was that they enjoyed treats and being special with opportunities to learn new skills related to their condition
- Bad things about diabetes were related to the pain of blood tests, sore fingers, loss of control and fears about the future
- Support was gained from parents, other adults, friends, peers and profes- sional staff

To put this information across to Gareth, Bannister (1996) implemented an on-going series of fun days to promote self-care in children aged ≥ 5 years, while Richmond (1998b) stated that children should be assessed for ability to self- inject at ~6 years of age. Although a bit young at present, Karen and Mark should provide Gareth with the opportunity to handle equipment and become familiar with aspects of diet and blood sugar testing. Amer (1999) states that young children are willing to ventilate and act out fears and anxieties, so information needs eliciting from Gareth.

Three months after diagnosis Karen and Mark would be eligible to claim disability living allowance to help with the extra costs incurred as a result of having a child with diabetes (McEvilly, 1997). They should also be made aware of the British Diabetic Association, which provides packs for parents, teachers, school canteen supervisors and cooks.

References

Amer, K. S. (1999). Children's adaptation to insulin dependant diabetes mellitus: a critical review of the literature. *Pediatric Nursing*, 25, 627–641.

American Diabetic Association (1997). Insulin administration. *Diabetes Care*, 20, S46–49.

Bannister, M. (1996). Promotion of diabetes self-care through play. *Professional Nurse*, 12, 109–112.

Brennan, A. (1996). Diabetes mellitus: a biomedical health education/promotion approach. *British Journal of Nursing*, 5, 1060–1064.

Challener, J. (1998a). Managing diabetes in children and adolescents: 1. *Professional Care of Mother and Child*, 8, 119–121.

Challener, J. (1998b). Managing diabetes in children and adolescents: 2. *Professional Care of Mother and Child*, 9, 11–13.

Cradock, S. (1995). Managing diabetes: knowledge for practice. *Nursing Times*, 91, S1–3.

Diabetic Control and Complications Trial Research Group (1994). Effects of Intensive diabetes treatment on the development and progression of long-term complications in adolescents with IDDM. *Journal of Paediatrics*, 125, 177–188.

Evans, D. D. M. (1994). *Special Tests*. London: Times Mirror International.

Faulkner, M. S., & Clark, F. S. (1998). Quality of life for parents of children and adolescents with type 1 diabetes. *Diabetes Educator*, 24, 721–727.

Gardner, N. (1998). Emotional and behavioural difficulties in children with diabetes: a controlled comparison with siblings and peers. *Child Care Health and Development*, 24, 115–128.

Harrop, M., Thornton, H., Woodhall, C., & Ratcliff, J. (1999). Improving paediatric diabetes care. *Nursing Standard*, 13, 38–43.

Hatton, D. L., Canam, C., Thorne, S., & Hughes, A. M. (1995). Parent's perceptions of caring for an infant or toddler with diabetes. *Journal of Advanced Nursing*, 22, 569–577.

Ingersoll, G. M., & Golden, M. P. (1995). The diabetic child in context: the child and family. In G. Kelner (ed.), *Childhood and Adolescent Diabetes Mellitus*. London: Chapman & Hall.

Kapit, W., Macey, R. I., & Meisami, E. (1998). *The Physiology Coloring Book*. New York: Harper & Row.

Landis, B. J. (1996). Uncertainty: spiritual well-being and psychological adjustment to chronic illness. *Issues in Mental Health Nursing*, 17, 267–271.

Lebovitz, H. E. (1995). Diabetic ketoacidosis. *Lancet*, 345, 767–772.

Lowes, L., & Davis, R. (1997). Focus on children's nursing. Minimising hospitalisation: children with newly diagnosed diabetes. *British Journal of Nursing*, 6, 28, 30–33.

Lowes, L., & Lyne, P. (1999). A normal life-style: parental stress and coping in childhood diabetes. *British Journal of Nursing*, 8, 133–139.

McEvilley, A. (1997). Childhood diabetes. *Paediatric Nursing*, 9, 29–33.

Miller, S. (1999). Hearing from children who have diabetes. *Journal of Child Health Care*, 3, 5–12.

Richmond, A. (1998). Childhood diabetes: dietary aspects. *Paediatric Nursing*, 10, 29–35.

Richmond, J. (1998). How important are the psychological aspects of diabetes? *Journal of Diabetes*, 2, 144–149.

Richmond, J. (1996). Effects of hypoglycaemia: patient's perceptions and experiences. *British Journal of Nursing*, 5, 1054–1059.

Selekman, J., Scofield, S., & Swenson-Brousell, C. (1999). Diabetes update in the pediatric population. *Pediatric Nursing*, 25, 666–669.

Shield, J. P., & Baum, J. B. (1998). Advances in childhood onset diabetes. *Archives of Diseases of Childhood*, 78, 391–394.

Weir, G. C., Nathan, D. M., & Singer, D. E. (1994). Standards of care [Technical Review]. *Diabetes Care*, 17, 1514–1522.

Wiklund, G., & Persson, B. (1999). Medical and psycho-social impact of acute infections in young patients. *Journal of Diabetes Nursing*, 3, 43–45, 48.

Yki-Jarvinen, H. (1994). The pathogenesis of NIDDM. *Lancet*, 343, 91–95.

Further reading

Watkins, P. J., & Drury, K. L. (1996). *Diabetes and Its Management*. Basingstoke: Blackwells.

Useful information

British Diabetic Association, 10 Queen Anne Street, London W1M 0BD, UK; tel.: 020 7323 1531.

Acute lymphoblastic leukaemia

Ruth Sadik

Catherine Summerville is the 3-year-old daughter of Simone and Jason. Until 2 weeks ago she was a happy lively child, full of fun and able to keep up with her older peers at nursery school. More recently, she has become very sleepy, appearing pale and clinging to Simone instead of running around as usual. Simone has also noticed that Catherine has more than her fair share of infections and is currently in the midst of her third ear infection. Last night as Simone went to check on Catherine before retiring for the night, she noticed that her daughter was 'burning up and very jittery'. On taking Cathy's temperature, she found it to be 39.6°C, and called the GP. A few hours later after the locum GP had examined Cathy and found bruising on her extremities and lower back, he suggested that their little girl be admitted to the local children's ward for further investigations. On arrival, blood was taken and Cathy and her mother settled into the ward.

After a long and stressful night in which Cathy was given IV antibiotics, the consultant informed Simone that she thought that Cathy had leukaemia and would need urgent referral to the regional children's oncology unit.

Following further tests and investigations, Cathy was diagnosed as having acute lymphoblastic leukaemia (ALL) and commenced on cytotoxic therapy in accordance with the current policy.

Question one: Outline the pathophysiology of acute lymphoblastic leukaemia (ALL).

15 minutes

Question two: Suggest appropriate ways of preparing Cathy for the interventions she is going to require during diagnosis and treatment.

25 minutes

Question three: Explain the potential side-effects that Cathy may experience from chemotherapy.

20 minutes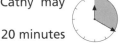

Question four: Explain the information that Simone and Jason will need to allow them to care for Cathy while at home.

15 minutes

Time Allocation: **1 hour 15 minutes**

Client profiles in nursing: child health

Answer to question one:

Outline the pathophysiology of acute lymphoblastic leukaemia (ALL).

Despite its rarity, cancer is the main cause of disease-related death in children aged 2–14 years (Richards *et al.*, 1998). Of all cancers, three-quarters are attributed to ALL, which affects children of all ages but predominates in boys aged 2–6 years (Hunt, 1995). According to the UK Children's Cancer Study Group (UKCCSG & Cancerbacup, 1999) > 400 new cases present every year in the UK.

ALL can be described as a malignant proliferation of lymphoblastic cells (one of the white cell line) (Figure 13.1), which comprise 30% or more of the bone marrow (Kanarek, 1998). In addition to replacing normal, mature erythrocytes, leukocytes and platelets, the immature 'blast' cells may also infiltrate the lymphatic nodes, spleen, liver and cerebrospinal fluid.

Most of Catherine's signs and symptoms (Table 13.1) arise as a result of leukaemic cell replacement of the bone marrow or blast infiltration to other sites.

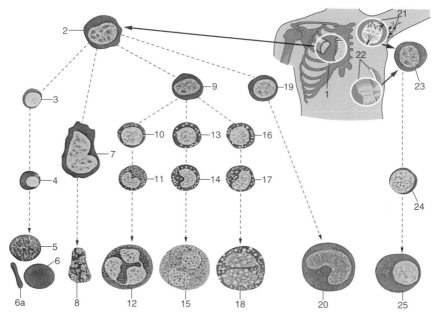

Figure 13.1. Development of blood cells. 1, Cross-section of rib and sternum showing red bone marrow; 2, haemohistioblast; 3, erythroblast; 4, normoblast; 5, reticulocyte; 6, adult red blood cell; 7, megakaryocyte; 8, platelet; 9, myeloblast; 10, neutrophilic myelocyte; 11, neutrophilic metamyelocyte; 12, polymorphonuclear neutrophile; 13, eosinophilic myelocyte; 14, eosinophilic metamyelocyte; 15, polymorphonuclear eosinophile; 16, basophilic myelocyte; 17, basophilic metamyelocyte; 18, polymorphonuclear basophile; 19, monoblast; 20, monocyte; 21, cross-section of an axillary lymph node showing lymphoid follicles; 22, cross-section of the spleen; 23, lymphoblast; 24, small lymphocyte; 25, large lymphocyte.

Table 13.1. Physiological effects of ALL.

	Physiological consequence	Effects on Catherine
Erythrocyte depletion	hypoxia due to decreased oxygen carrying capacity	anaemia, dyspnoea, pallor, lethargy
Leukocyte depletion	immune response delayed or absent	recurrent infections
Platelet depletion	thrombolytic response decreases	bruising either spontaneously or on slight pressure, haemorrhage
Hepatosplenic infiltration	replacement of normal cells with abnormal blast cells	enlargement of organs, potential loss of function
Bone marrow infiltration	expansion of intramedullary lumen	bone and joint pain, limping, abnormal positioning

The cause of ALL remains unknown; however, various factors have been identified as predisposing to its development. According to Campbell (1996), these are ionizing radiation, familial predisposition and chromosomal abnormalities such as Down's syndrome, while the Leukaemia Research Fund (1997) identified a rare reaction to common infectious agents and perinatal exposure to chemicals or electromagnetic fields.

Answer to question two:
Suggest appropriate ways of preparing Cathy for the interventions she is going to require during diagnosis and treatment.

Cathy and her parents will need educating about the disease and its treatments, as the more informed they are the more likely they are to anticipate and manage undesirable side-effects.

Most of the tests, investigations and treatments that Cathy requires may be repetitive, invasive and unpleasant. The tests, investigations and treatments for ALL are:

- X-rays
- CT (computed tomographic) scan
- MRI (magnetic resonance imaging)
- Lumbar puncture (LP)
- Bone marrow aspiration (BMA)
- Blood samples
- Central venous catheter (long line): wound dressing and changing

To lessen the impact, the multidisciplinary team needs to coordinate their input.

Supportive care will involve:

- IV feeding if oral intake becomes too painful
- Blood transfusion depending on Catherine's blood results
- Infection prevention: antibiotics may be given
- Protective isolation where Cathy may be nursed in a single room. Everyone having contact with Cathy will be free of infections such as coughs and colds, wash their hands and adopt universal precautions

Communication with children so young, or anxious parents, may be difficult for the nurse who could find herself faced by questions and dilemmas which she is ill-equipped to answer (May, 1999). Young children have a limited ability to communicate familiar needs, and expressing anxieties and fears are even more difficult.

Brennan (1994) identified that children of Cathy's age frequently act out their fears and fantasies in distressed and destructive behaviours. An inability to understand complex concepts and verbal explanations culminates in fears of bodily distortion, mutilation or annihilation (Brennan, 1994).

Young childrens' coping mechanisms differ from adults in that they have an increased perception of threat from misunderstanding the stressful event. They lack experience or knowledge of potential resources both internal and external that they can bring to the situation and even when they have these skills, they often lack the ability to implement them effectively. Nurses, therefore, need to be aware of Catherine's cognitive, physical and communication skill level. May (1999) identified strategies such as drawing, humour, music, storytelling as being useful adjuncts; however, Heiney (1991) outlined three distinct phases that Catherine will need help mastering to allow her to cope with potential trauma:

- Anticipation of and preparation for the event
- Actual event
- Aftermath that appears to be the most traumatic period for the child and carers and 'may involve pain, restricted movement, anxiety about results and lingering emotional trauma' (Heiney, 1991: 20)

Doverty (1992) explored the usefulness of drama-play in enabling Catherine to adjust to stress and anxiety. He highlighted the use of play in making therapeutic activities fun. Involving Simone and Jason in ascertaining Catherine's favourite play activities, increases their feelings of involvement and control. Play is a natural activity for children, which allows them to explore and express thoughts and feelings. When planning play activities consideration should be given to creating time for planned therapeutic play in conjunction with normal unstructured activities. Medical play can involve the use of dolls, puppets, games and stories and can be used to prepare Catherine. One strategy (Stephens *et al.*, 1999) involves:

- Stress immunisation and desensitisation: involves a series of preparatory sessions where the child is introduced to increasingly stressful events before the actual event. The child is taught coping skills and has their fears addressed
- Teaching coping skills: may include relaxation, imagery and distraction, thought stopping and cognitive restructuring
- Stress-point preparation: provides information regarding the anticipated event, providing time and help to prepare a response. Emotional and physical support would be maintained throughout all interventions for both Cathy and her parents to ensure the least traumatic outcome for all concerned

In summary, members of the multiprofessional team can help Cathy deal with the barrage of tests, investigations and treatments. The strategies to help Cathy cope are:

- Individualized care based on age, experience, personality and level of development
- Verbal and tactile communication throughout the procedure with in-built debriefing time
- Acknowledgement of feelings
- Normalization of responses
- Soft comforting sounds
- Offering choice to increase the sense of control
- Outline what Cathy should expect and what adults will expect of her
- Identify what part Simone and Jason will play in coaching Cathy through the procedure

Answer to question three:
Explain the potential side-effects that Cathy may experience from chemotherapy.

Catherine has a 70% chance of cure with the current medical treatment for ALL (Smith *et al.*, 1996). It combines treatment modalities of multi-agent chemo-therapy with or without central nervous system (CNS) radiation, and involves the introduction of chemical agents that destroy normal as well as malignant cells. This accounts for the range of toxic effects experienced by Cathy. The major classes of cytotoxic drugs likely to be used in Cathy's treatment are given in Table 13.2.

As malignant cells replicate at a greater speed than non-malignant cells treatment is targeted at preventing cell division. The drugs used are mainly non-specific in action and so also affect rapidly dividing normal cells such as those found in the mucous membrane of the mouth and gastrointestinal system, hair and skin follicles, and bone marrow. These effects are usually reversible once treatment stops.

Table 13.2. Cytotoxic drugs used in lymphoblastic leukaemia.

Classification	Action	Drug	Side-effects	Nursing implications
Alkylating	interfere with DNA replication	cyclophosphamide	urinary tract haemorrhage, cardio-myopathy, alopecia, skin rashes and nausea	high fluid intake based on Catherine's age and weight test all urine for blood, glucose and pH fluid balance record
		sodium mercaptoethane sulphate (mesna)	given to limit toxicity of above	
Anthracycline antibiotics	bind with DNA to prevent replication and transcription	daunorubicin	bone marrow suppression, alopecia, phlebitis, nausea and vomiting, diarrhoea, red urine, rash, cardiotoxicity	observe stools, ECG monitoring, warn of red urine for up to 12 days
		doxorubicin	similar but no red urine	
Epipodo-phyllotoxins	inhibits topoisomerase II during replication and transcription	etoposide	hypotension if infused rapidly, alopecia, oral ulceration, anaphylactic reactions occur rarely	temperature, pulse, respiration and blood pressure monitoring
Vinca alkaloids	block the formation of the mitotic spindle	vincristine	abdominal, jaw bone and joint pain, peripheral neuropathy, constipation	observe for signs of neurotoxicity stool chart and consider stool softeners
Corticosteroids		prednisolone	immunosuppression, peptic ulceration, dyspepsia, sodium and water retention, hypertension, growth suppression, hirsutism, increased appetite, precipitation of diabetes, glaucoma, bruising and impaired healing	regular testing of urine, blood pressure observe skin for loss of integrity, hair growth monitor height, weight, bone age, vision
Antineoplastic	miscellaneous	asparaginase	anaphylactic reaction, weight loss, neurotoxicity, fever, clotting disturbances, blood glucose disturbance, renal and liver dysfunction, pancreatitis	resuscitative measures in case of anaphylaxis daily weight
Antimetabolites	prevent the uptake of chemicals essential to cell division	methotrexate (deprives cell of folic acid)	renal damage, severe systemic toxicity, mouth ulcers	IV hydration and alkalization 6 h before administration. Test all urine to pH 7–8
		folinic acid (calcium leucovorin rescue)	to counteract effects	
		cytarabine	bone marrow depressant, conjunctivitis, liver damage, gut toxicity, oral ulceration	observe for signs of anaemia, infection, bruising, bleeding, sore eyes, jaundice and oral ulceration
		mercaptopurine (interferes with nucleic acid)	rare but may include bone marrow suppression, liver damage	

Answer to question four:
Explain the information that Simone and Jason will need to allow them to care for Cathy while at home.

When Catherine's white cell, especially her neutrophil count has reached normal limits she will be allowed home.

Caring for the family with a child undergoing treatment for cancer involves a multi-agency approach, involving cooperation between the local district general hospital, the specialist regional centre and community providers. Jason and Simone should be familiar with the agencies involved in their care before discharge and should expect to liaise, on a regular basis with some of the following:

- Doctors and nurses specialized in the care of children with cancer
- Children's community nurses
- Play specialist
- Health visitor
- GP
- Haematologist
- Dietician
- Radiographer and radiologist
- Social worker
- Psychologist
- Pharmacist
- Pathologist

These personnel might be available from either or both the regional and local hospitals involved in sharing the care of Catherine and her family.

The role of the children's nurse in working with parents such as Simone and Jason is mainly supportive education. Catherine's parents should be helped to understand the various therapies, prevention and management of possible side-effects and observation for any late effects of therapy.

However, before they can begin to become involved in Catherine's care they should be assisted in dealing constructively with their own emotional turmoil. This may include counselling, clear concise information about diagnosis and clarification of their role in Catherine's care. Self-help groups or organizations such as Cancerbacup or Leukaemia Busters can help them explore how to inform Catherine and other family members.

They will also need an awareness of the way in which Catherine may respond to being ill, especially in relation to regressive behaviour and the effects this may have on themselves and the extended family. They need to be sure of the role they can both play in discipline, and need explicitly to discuss how they feel about imposing limits on Cathy's behaviour at this vulnerable time. Cathy should continue to attend the nursery as it will assist in regaining normalization of her daily routine, helps develop sense of independence and reinforces that her parents consistently come back and get her.

At a practical level they will want procedural information related to radio-therapy, central venous catheter care, infection control and nutrition.

Specific need will depend on both Cathy and her parents' response to the illness, treatment and outcomes. Regardless of this, the nurse's role continues to be one of collaboration and empowerment.

References

Brennan, A. (1994). Caring for children during procedures: a review of the literature. *Pediatric Nursing*, 20, 451–458, 460–461.

Campbell, K. (1996). Lymphoblastic leukaemia: classification and treatment. *Nursing Times*, 93, 31–32.

Doverty, N. (1992). Therapeutic use of play in hospital. *British Journal of Nursing*, 1, 77–81.

Heiney, S. P. (1991). Helping children through painful procedures. *American Journal of Nursing*, 91, 20–24.

Hunt, J. (1995). Childhood leukaemia. *Paediatric Nursing*, 7, 29–36.

Kanarek, R. (1998). Facing the challenge of childhood leukemia. *American Journal of Nursing*, 98, 42–47.

Leukaemia Research Fund (1997). Acute leukaemia in children [http://leukaemia.demon.co.uk].

May, L. (1999). 'I've got tummy ache in my head'. Communicating with sick children. *Paediatric Nursing*, 11, 21–23.

Richards, S., Burrett, J., Hann, I., Chessles, J., Hill, F., & Bailey, C. (1998). Improved survival with early intensification: combined results from the Medical Research Council childhood ALL randomised trials, UKALL X and UKALL XI. *Leukaemia*, 12, 1031–1036.

Rossen, B. E., & McKeeven, P. D. (1996). The behavior of pre-schoolers during and after brief surgical hospitalization. *Issues in Comprehensive Pediatric Nursing*, 19, 121–133.

Smith, M., Arthur, D., & Camitta, B. (1996). Uniform approach to risk classification and treatment assignment for children with acute lymphoblastic leukemia and a slow response to initial treatment. *Journal of Clinical Oncology*, 14, 18–24.

Stephens, B. K., Barkey, M. E., & Hall, H. R. (1999). Techniques to comfort children during stressful procedures. *Accident and Emergency Nursing*, 7, 226–236.

UK Children's Cancer Study Group & Cancerbacup (1999). *A Parent's Guide to Children's Cancers*. London: UKCCSG & Cancerbacup.

Further reading

Audit Commission (1993). *Children First: A Study of Hospital Services*. London: HMSO.

Casey, G. (1999). Wound management in children. *Paediatric Nursing*, 11, 39–45.

Cook, N. (1999). Central venous catheters: preventing infection and occlusion. *British Journal of Nursing*, 8, 980–989.

Corbett, A. (1997). Mouth care and chemotherapy. *Paediatric Nursing*, 9, 19–21.

Reid, U. (1997). Stigma of hair loss after chemotherapy. *Paediatric Nursing*, 9, 16–18.

Shelley, P. (1995). Contact a family. *Paediatric Nursing*, 7, 6–8.

Wilson, C. J. (1999). Parental preparation of children for routine physical examination. *Journal of Pediatric Nursing: Nursing Care of Children and Families*, 14, 329–335.

Useful information

http://cancernet.nci.gov/clinpdqq
http://imsdd.meb.uni-bonn.de/cancernet
http://leukaemia.demon.co.uk
http://oncolink.upenn.edu
http://www.noah.cuny.edu/cancer
http://www.penlex.org.uk/lbfacts.html

Strabismus

Gill Campbell

> Colin Clark is a 4-year-old boy who has been under observation by the Eye Department at his local hospital with myopia (short-sightedness) since he was 10 months old. It has become apparent over the past year that Colin has a squint (strabismus) in his left eye, which is directly attributable to myopia. As this is being corrected with prescription spectacles, and Colin starts school in 3 months time, it is now deemed appropriate to correct this eye muscle imbalance. This will help both to prevent amblyopia ('lazy eye') developing and to stop children making fun of him.
>
> Colin's local hospital performs strabismus surgery on a daycase basis, and he and his father, Geoff, are invited to attend a preclerking session 3 days before admission. They are informed that Colin will require a left lateral rectus resection and a medial rectus recession.

Question one: Draw a diagram of the eye, identifying the six extrinsic muscles and give their functions.

20 minutes

Question two: Explain the care and management that Colin will need during the postoperative period.

20 minutes

Time Allowance: **40 minutes**

Answer to question one:
Draw a diagram of the eye, identifying the six extrinsic muscles and give their functions.

The six muscles move the eye inwards, outwards, upwards and downwards (Figure 14.1). The lateral rectus moves the eyeball outwards, while inward movement is brought about by the medial rectus. The muscle that controls upward movement of the eyeball is the superior rectus, while the inferior rectus moves the eyeball downwards. The superior oblique muscle moves the eye downwards and out, while it is moved upwards and out by the inferior oblique (Brooker, 1998).

As Colin requires a left lateral rectus resection and a medial rectus recession, this means that pre-operatively Colin's left eye will be being pulled in the mid line towards his nose.

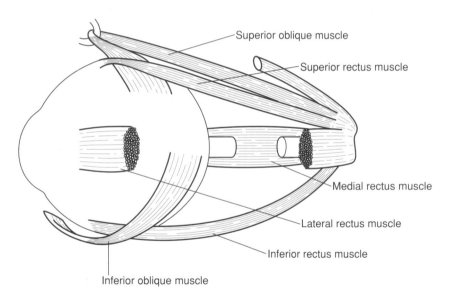

Figure 14.1. Extrinsic muscles of the eye.

Answer to question two:
Explain the care and management that Colin will need during the postoperative period.

As soon as Colin returns to the care of the nurses he should have his airway assessed for patency and his cough reflex checked. Baseline observations of his pulse, respirations, BP and temperature should be taken (Campbell & Glasper, 1995), and continued on a regular basis until Colin is fully awake and his vital signs are stable. Pain following correction of strabismus is usually minimal but assessment (see Profile 23, Melanie Court) should be commenced as soon as Colin returns to the ward and he should be actively involved as soon as he is able. Pain relief should be administered as prescribed. Anti-emetics are frequently prescribed for children following strabismus surgery and these should be administered regularly. Colin may suffer from post-operative vomiting as this is known to occur in > 33% of children > 2 years of age undergoing this type of surgery (Allen *et al.*, 1998). This is possibly caused by the effect of an oculocardiac reflex (OCR) on the vomiting centre in the medulla, which can occur during eye surgery as part of a vasovagal response (Allen *et al.*, 1998). Colin should start drinking fluids slowly to decrease the risk of vomiting.

Urine output should be monitored as it is necessary to establish that urine retention is not occurring (Campbell & Glasper, 1995). Urinary retention may occur as a side-effect of anaesthetic gases by relaxing the muscle tone of the bladder (Moules & Ramsay, 1998). Retention may also occur by the body responding to the stress of surgery. Antidiuretic hormone (ADH) is produced in the anterior lobe of the pituitary gland in increased quantities in response to this stress. ADH then acts on the renal tubules, which increases their permeability. The effect of this is to reduce or eliminate water excretion (Campbell & Glasper, 1995; Moules & Ramsay, 1998).

Colin will need to receive antibiotic eye drops (e.g. chloramphenicol) to prevent infection and steroid eye drops (e.g. prednisolone) to reduce inflam-mation. These will be administered four times daily and will commence 4–24 h postoperatively dependent on the prescription.

It is important that Colin is fully stable before discharge. Generally, he would not be permitted to be discharged until he had both eaten and drunk, and had passed urine. Day surgery reduces the anxieties a child may have about being away from home, but this might increase the responsibilities for the family (Ireland & Rushforth, 1998). It is, therefore, important for the nurse to communicate with the family to ensure that they are happy for Colin to be discharged to their care and are aware of who to turn to for help if they have any concerns.

References

Allen, L. E., Sudesh, S., Sandramouli, S., Cooper, G., McFarlane, D., & Willshaw, H. E. (1998). The association between the oculocardiac reflex and post-operative vomiting in children undergoing strabismus surgery. *Eye*, 12, 193–196.

Brooker, C. (1998). *Human Structure and Function*. London: Mosby.

Campbell, S., & Glasper, E. A. (eds) (1995). *Whaley and Wong's Children's Nursing*. London: Mosby.

Ireland, L., & Rushforth, H. (1998). Day-care – in whose best interests? *Paediatric Nursing*, 10, 15–19.

Further reading

American Academy of Ophthalmology (1994). Strabismus: etiology, diagnosis, and treatment. *Journal of Ophthalmic Nursing and Technology*, 13, 121–123.

Anon. (1999, accessed 25 July 2000). Crossed eyes of wall eye (strabismus) and lazy eye (amblyopia) [http://onhealth.com/conditions/resource/conditions/item%2C52107.as].

Anon. (n.d., accessed 25 July 2000). Strabismus [http://homepages.iol.ie/~rhmajor/strab.HTM].

Department of Health (1998, accessed 27 July 2000). Implications of day case surgery [http://www.doh.gov.uk/ntrd/rd/psi/priority/first/14.htm].

Hodge, D. (ed.) (1999). *Day Surgery: A Nursing Approach*. Edinburgh: Churchill Livingstone.

Montgomery, C. (1997). Early eye care checks for children. *Practice Nurse*, 14, 246–249.

Moorfields Eye Hospital NHS Trust (n.d., accessed 25 July 2000). Eyes in focus insight into squint (strabismus) [http://www.moorfields.org.uk/ef-squint.htm].

Olitsky, S. E., & Nelson, L. B. (1998). Common ophthalmologic concerns in infants and children. *Pediatric Clinics of North America*, 45, 993–1012.

Winter-Griffith, H. (1995, accessed 27 July 2000). Strabismus surgery [http://www.thriveonline.com/health/Library/surgery/surgery6.1htm].

Seven-year-old with depression

Lucy Davies and Ruth Sadik

Jack Hunter is a 7-year-old Caucasian boy. He lives at home with his mother Helen, father Paul and sisters Elizabeth and Kate, aged 11 and 5 respectively.

Jack has been admitted to the local children's ward following a 3-month history of acute stomach pains. All appropriate tests have been conducted and no apparent pathological cause has been found to explain his stomach-ache.

His teachers at school report that during his intermittent attendance he had been inattentive and appeared to be distracted. His schoolwork had deteriorated over the past 3 months and he had lost interest in activities that he used to enjoy, like football. His teachers also noticed that Jack was isolating himself from his peers, a factor agreed with by Jack's parents as he no longer had friends round to the house to play.

Jack has complained of not being able to sleep, and he says that he is often tired on waking and during the day. His appetite has been poor, he picks at food and has failed to put any weight on over the 3 months. He looks underweight, which is confirmed when he is weighed on admission and found to be the same weight he was 2 years ago, 23 kg.

His mother reports that her son has been more irritable than usual, particularly with his younger sister, towards whom he is worryingly aggressive. She also says that Jack is constantly blaming himself for things that go wrong. He has even felt responsible for his father's bad moods, saying that he makes them happen because he is naughty. The children's psychiatrist is asked to see Jack, and diagnoses him as being depressed.

Question one: Explain Jack's signs and symptoms of depression.

20 minutes

Question two: Outline the nursing interventions that would be helpful to Jack and his family.

30 minutes

Time Allocation: **50 minutes**

Answer to question one:
Explain Jack's signs and symptoms of depression.

There are two main classification systems of mental health disorders that are referred to widely in specialised texts on mental health. Both the Diagnostic and Statistical Manual of Mental Disorders (DSM)-IV (Frances, 1994) and the International Classification of Diseases (ICD)-10 (World Health Organisation, 1992) identify that over time a number of the following symptoms must be present and consistent for at least 2 weeks and must occur almost every day for a diagnosis of depression to be made. These are:

- Either subjectively (complaining of feeling sad) or objectively (observation by others) a depressed mood. In young children this may present as excessive irritability
- Lack of interest or pleasure in all or most of the usual activities
- Increase or decrease in appetite where weight is lost or gained. This may be measured in children as failure to meet expected weight gains
- Insomnia (inability to sleep) or hypersomnia (sleeping more than usual and during the day)
- Objective perception of psychomotor retardation or agitation
- Feeling of tiredness or lack of energy
- Complaining of feeling worthless
- Inability to concentrate properly accompanied by indecision
- Recurrent thoughts of death, with ideas of how to commit it or an actual attempt
- Symptoms cause 'clinically significant distress or impairment in social occupational or other important areas of functioning'
- Symptoms are not present because of drug (mis)use or a medical condition
- Symptoms cannot be attributed to a recent (within 2 months) bereavement
- Symptoms do not meet the criterion for 'a mixed episode', that is they are not attributable to an already existing and diagnosable illness (Frances, 1994: 327)

Factors that might contribute to depression are (Barker, 1995; Armstrong, 1996):

- Positive parental history of affective disorder – may be environmental or genetic
- Inconsistent discipline
- Separation from attachment figure through bereavement, divorce, hospitalisation
- Learned helplessness (victim mentality)
- Biochemical dysfunction
- Secondary phenomenon to other disorders
- Side-effect of medications such as steroids
- Side-effect of street drugs such as cocaine

The incidence rate of affective (mood) disorders among children aged 14–17 years is estimated to be ~4%, with girls being more likely to suffer than boys (Whitaker *et al.*, 1990, Weaver, 1995). However, before puberty the rate is much lower and it predominates in boys (Whitaker *et al.*, 1990; Harrington, 1994). Barker (1995) noted that pre-pubertal depression is often associated with concurrent difficulties such as poor scholarly performance, or a family history of alcoholism or anti-social behaviour.

Like Jack, it is quite common for depressed school-aged children to somatise their experience of depression, frequently complaining of stomach-ache (Barker, 1995; Oakley and Potter, 1997). It has also been noted (Oakley and Potter, 1997) that depressed children experience poor sleep patterns and impaired concentration. At school this might lead to poorer performance, notably an unwillingness to undertake tasks such as writing and drawing. They may also resist joining in with participatory games, stating that they 'can't'.

Depression has only recently been recognised in young children as it can be missed or masked by the presentation of the physical condition. However, the standardisation of clinical assessment and a willingness on the part of clinicians to ask children about their experiences rather than relying mainly on the reports of significant adults has significantly improved recognition (Weaver, 1995). Sharman (1997) cautioned, however, that most of the assessment tools are currently devised for adult clients and may not be appropriate for use with children and advises that depressive-like phenomena must be considered in the light of normal child development. While it is unusual to see suicidal behaviour in children < 12 years, imaginary ideas and plans about suicide are commonly expressed (Sharman, 1997). It cannot be over emphasised that referral to the specialist child and family mental health service should be done as early as possible in the assessment and treatment of Jack.

Client profiles in nursing: child health

Answer to question two:
Outline the nursing interventions that would be helpful to Jack and his family.

The goals of care will have been determined by a member of the mental health team in collaboration with both Jack and his parents. If Jack's depression is thought to be mild, encouraging his family to participate positively in sympathetic discussions with him, while empowering Jack to cope with any stressful situations in his life has been reported (Harrington, 1994) as having a significant impact on lightening the child's mood. Family involvement is the cornerstone of care as it is the family that has the responsibility of reaching the goals of treatment.

Elizabeth and Kate are both old enough to be involved in Jack's management. However, sibling involvement is often dependent on the data gleaned, ages of siblings and parental wishes. Sharman (1997) suggested a four-point plan of intervention that might be useful for Jack and his family:

- Child's safety
    - environment: including points such as access to windows, drugs, electricity or sharp implements
    - supervision: it is essential to assess the level of supervision that Jack would require to keep him safe. He may need one-to-one supervision where he is under constant observation or regular supervision where the nursing staff would check on him every 15 min. The aim is to ensure that Jack has minimal opportunity to harm himself and may be reassured by the presence of a responsible adult
    - contract: a set of firm rules drawn up with the agreement of both Jack and the nursing staff. While accepting that Jack has a right to express all emotions, it is useful to reinforce positive behaviour and dissuade negative behaviour such as self-harm or self-neglect
- Individual work: a single nurse per shift should be identified as Jack's key nurse. This enables him to develop a relationship or therapeutic alliance with as few individuals as possible. In the case of children with mental health problems, the value of the therapeutic relationship cannot be underestimated, a trusting relationship will enable Jack to express any thoughts and feelings in a safe and appropriate way. There are tools that can be helpful in the development of the relationship. An example might be a feelings thermometer that would allow Jack to grade feelings in terms of hot or cold, or if appropriate he could be asked to keep a diary. This would help to formulate patterns of events and give Jack a feeling of being in control. Presenting him with simply drawn faces with easy-to-recognise expressions such as sad, happy and sleepy can also help Jack to express how he feels
- Other strategies for building self-esteem, but which would not be carried out by children's nurses without the required qualification, are group and family therapy, individual psychoanalytical therapy and, the most successful of all with depressed children (Rutter *et al.*, 1994), cognitive-behavioural therapy. As Jack may be experiencing anxiety as part of his depression, it can be useful to introduce relaxation techniques. Encouraging him to manage his

breathing in a soothing pattern and perhaps introducing tapes or music may also benefit him. Depressed adults and children will frequently misinterpret everyday events around them, for example seeing another difficulty as something for which they are directly responsible. This could explain Jack's feeling of responsibility for his father's bad moods. The nursing staff can use reframing techniques, where they help Jack to reframe experiences by putting a more realistic interpretation on the events and enable him to see them in a more positive light

- Improving self-esteem: Sharman (1997) suggested that helping Jack to improve his self-esteem underpins all interventions offered to him. Examples of strategies to help Jack are:
  - at bed-time, reviewing his accomplishments of the day, which may help to put a positive focus on his behaviours
  - drawing an outline of a boy's body with positive statements attached to different parts might help in bringing out more positive statements from Jack
  - supporting Jack in drawing a 'road map' of his past and future may help in demonstrating what he has, and can achieve
  - Weaver (1995) agreed with much of what Sharman suggested, but he also stressed the role of the family in facilitating Jack's care. He introduced the possibility of psychotropic medication in Jack's treatment although he identifies that this should be as a final resort and as an area to be explored by specialists in the mental health field as many of these drugs are not licensed for use with children in the UK. Given, however, that they are relatively safe in overdose, Weaver (1995) advocates the use of serotonin-specific drugs such as fluoxitine (Prozac), as opposed to the older tricyclic type of antidepressant medication. Hampshire (1998) reported on the use of Prozac with children in the UK and commented that it is currently the treatment of choice with ~50 children.

Regardless of the mode of treatment, it is unclear what the outcomes of depressive disorders in childhood are (Harrington, 1994; Armstrong, 1996). However, Harrington (1994) cited several papers that indicate that depressive episodes are highly likely to recur, and often continue into adult life. It is for this reason that children like Jack often stay on the case-load of the psychiatric service for several years.

References

Armstrong, K. (1996). Childhood depression. *Practice Nurse*, 11, 243, 245–247.
Barker, P. J. (1995). *Basic Child Psychiatry*. Oxford: Blackwells.
Frances, A. (ed.) (1994). *Diagnostic and Statistical Manual of Mental Disorders*, 4th edn. Washington, DC: American Psychiatric Association.
Hampshire, M. (1998). The Prozac children. *Nursing Times*, 94, 12–13.
Harrington, R. (1994). Affective disorders. In M. Rutter, R. Taylor, & L. Hersov (eds), *Child and Adolescent Psychiatry* (330–345). Oxford: Blackwells.
Oakley, K., & Potter, C. (1997). *Psychiatric Primary Care*. London: Baillière Tindall.
Rutter, M., Taylor, R., & Hersov, L. (eds) (1994). *Child and Adolescent Psychiatry*. Oxford: Blackwells.
Sharman, W. (1997). *Children and Adolescents with Mental Health Problems*. London: Baillière Tindall.

Weaver, A. (1995). Childhood depression. *Maternal and Child Health*, 20, 192–198.

Whitaker, A., Johnson, J., Shaffer, D., Rapoport, J. L., Kalikow, K., Walsh, B. T., Davies, M., Braiaman, S., & Dolinsky, A. (1990). Uncommon troubles in young people. *Archives of General Psychiatry*, 47, 487–496.

World Health Organisation (1992). Tenth Revision of the international classification of diseases. Chapter V. (F): Mental and Behavioural Disorder. *Clinical Descriptions and Diagnostic Guidelines*. Geneva: WHO.

Further reading

Goodman, R. (ed.) (1997). *Child Psychiatry*. Oxford: Blackwells.

Goodyer, I (ed.) (1995). *The Depressed Child and Adolescent Developmental and Clinical Perspectives*. Cambridge: Cambridge University Press.

Payne, B. J., & Range, L. M. (1996). Family environment, attitudes toward life and death, depression and suicidality in elementary-school children. *Death Studies*, 20, 481–494.

Pankhurst, L. (1997). Distress signals. *Open Mind*, 86, 8–9.

Epilepsy

Tessa Horlock

Jamie is a 7-year-old boy who lives with his parents Sue and John and his 10-year-old brother, Mark. He is an active child who enjoys playing football with his sibling. He is also a keen swimmer, and has been having swimming lessons since he was 4 years of age. Jamie hopes that one day he will swim for his country.

Jamie started school when he was 4 years old and got on very well, being in the top half of his class. He is a sociable boy with many friends.

Recently, Jamie's parents had noticed that he appeared to be daydreaming a lot and they found it increasingly difficult to attract his attention on these occasions. His teacher, Miss Hurst, had also noticed that Jamie was not as attentive as normal and was concerned that his schoolwork might suffer.

Jamie's mother took him to see their GP, who told her that he suspected that Jamie might have a form of epilepsy. The GP referred them to a paediatrician at their local hospital.

Jamie and his parents attend their appointment with the paediatrician who, following investigation, diagnoses Jamie as having absence epilepsy. He prescribed sodium valproate, an anti-epileptic medication.

Jamie's parents are understandably concerned about the cause of his epilepsy; and say they do not know anyone with the condition. They would like to know more about the diagnosis and treatment. They and Jamie are given the opportunity to discuss these issues with a nurse.

Question one: Outline the common causes of epilepsy and describe the presentation of absence seizures.

20 minutes

Question two: Discuss the way that you would explain Jamie's seizures to him and his family to reassure them.

15 minutes

Question three: What investigations are likely to be undertaken to aid Jamie's diagnosis?

10 minutes

Question four: Outline the aims of Jamie's treatment and the common side-effects of sodium valproate.

15 minutes

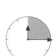

Question five: Briefly explain to Jamie and his parents some of the safety issues that need to be considered for a child with seizures.

15 minutes

Time Allocation: **1 hour 15 minutes**

Answer to question one:
Outline the common causes of epilepsy and describe the presentation of absence seizures.

Epilepsy is diagnosed when someone has largely unprovoked recurrent seizures. Such seizures are caused by abnormal excitability of the neurones in the brain (Appleton & Gibbs, 1995). It affects ~420 000 people in the UK; ~1:130 people, with the cause being unknown in about six of 10 people (BEA, 1999). In cases where a cause can be established, these vary depending on the age of the child at presentation (Table 16.1) (Hopkins & Appleton, 1996).

Table 16.1. Causes of epilepsy in childhood.

Newborn	Infant	Child
Anoxia at birth	genetic disorders,	genetic disorders
Trauma at birth	e.g. lipidosis	congenital abnormalities
Infectious diseases, e.g. meningitis	febrile convulsions	trauma
Acquired metabolic disease,	infectious diseases	tumours
e.g. hypoglycaemia		infectious diseases

There are many types of epilepsy, so it is important that a correct diagnosis is made before any treatment is commenced. It is suspected that Jamie has absence epilepsy and may be experiencing a brief lapse in consciousness. During this time he will normally stop what he is doing and stare. His head may drop forward and he may flutter his eyelids. The onset and termination of absence seizures is usually abrupt and they often go unnoticed, as the child will usually return to what they were doing before the seizure occurred (Kempthorne & Johnson, 1994). Jamie is also unlikely to remember his seizures and could have several during one day (Hopkins & Appleton, 1996).

Answer to question two:
Discuss the way that you would explain Jamie's seizures to him and his family to reassure them.

Jamie and his family are likely to be very anxious about the new diagnosis, so reassurance is going to be a large part of any explanations given. It is important to give Mr and Mrs Harley clear and concise information about the seizures that Jamie is having at the time of his diagnosis, and to be positive about his condition. Most children with epilepsy have the normal range of abilities as those of other children without the condition, so his intelligence is unlikely to be affected (BEA, 1999). The importance of taking medication should be emphasised and the long-term outlook for Jamie should be explained. In Jamie's case, the outlook is quite good as in many cases the seizures remit (Appleton & Gibbs, 1995).

Jamie should also have his seizures explained to him in a language he will understand. Children have vivid imaginations so it is important to prevent any fears and anxieties (BEA, 1999). It is likely that Jamie will have many questions in the future so it is important to ensure that his parents are adequately informed so that they can answer them.

Answer to question three:
What investigations are likely to be undertaken to aid Jamie's diagnosis?

Referral to a paediatrician or a consultant specialising in epilepsy is very important if the GP suspects that a child might have epilepsy. Several tests are likely to take place, but most importantly a detailed history should be taken, including information such as eyewitness accounts of seizures, general health status, childhood development and a family history of seizures or epilepsy. A full neurological examination should take place and information should be sought on any previous neurological problems such as head injuries or meningitis (Taylor, 1996).

Blood and urine analysis should be carried out to help identify a cause for the epilepsy. The other most likely investigation will be an electroencephalogram (EEG). This records the presence of normal and abnormal electrical activity in the brain (Lanfear & Fielding, 1998). This then helps to indicate the focus and type of epilepsy. Other tests carried out may include brain scans, e.g. magnetic resonance imaging (MRI) and computed tomography (CT), which can identify structural abnormalities within the brain that may be causing the epilepsy (Russell, 1996).

Answer to question four:
Outline the aims of Jamie's treatment and the common side-effects of sodium valproate.

The aims of the treatment of epilepsy with medication is to try and control seizures with the minimum of side-effects from the drug that they are taking (Mangan *et al.*, 1994a, b). The aim is to try and stop seizures altogether, so combinations of drugs may be required for good control of seizures, which will occur in 75–80% of people (Lanfear & Fielding, 1998).

For Jamie, the first line treatment will be sodium valproate, which is effective in controlling absence seizures (Appleton & Gibbs, 1995). All anti-epileptic medications have recognised side-effects, these fall into three groups. First, dose-related side-effects, that is when the dose given is too high. These include tremor, sedation and increased appetite. The second group is allergic reactions to the drug that include stomach irritation and inflammation of the liver and pancreas. The third group is related to chronic use of the drug, the most common being weight gain, alopecia and a low platelet count in the blood (Hopkins & Appleton, 1996).

Answer to question five:
Briefly explain to Jamie and his parents some of the safety issues that need to be considered for a child who has seizures.

Children with epilepsy should be encourage to lead as normal a life as possible. Having epilepsy is probably going to have long-term implications in their life as they grow older. It is, therefore, important that they continue to enjoy their childhood. Maintaining safety is an important issue in all children, but particularly in those with epilepsy, and consideration should be given to continued participation in activities that could be dangerous if a seizure occurred. Jamie should continue to swim but should always be supervised by someone who knows what to do in the event of a seizure (Mangan *et al.*, 1994a, b). Safety in the home and garden should be considered, particularly anything involving water, or other dangers around the home, like fires and cookers. The school needs to be informed of the type of seizures that Jamie has so that it can continue to observe him and ensure his safety.

References

Appleton, R., & Gibbs, J. (1995). *Epilepsy in Childhood and Adolescence*. London: Martin Dunitz.

British Epilepsy Association. (1999, accessed 1 August 2000). Information [http://www.epilepsy.org.uk].

Hopkins, A., & Appleton, R. (1996). *Epilepsy. The Facts*. Oxford: Oxford University Press.

Kempthorne, A., & Johnson, J. (1994). Epilepsy in childhood. *Paediatric Nursing*, 6, 30–33.

Lanfear J., & Fielding, A. (1994). The child/young person with epilepsy. *Paediatric Nursing*, 10, 29–36.

Mangan, P., Kershaw, B., & Lewis, K. (1994a). Epilepsy revision notes. *Nursing Times*, 90, 9–14.

Mangan, P., Kershaw, B., & Lewis, K. (1994b). Epilepsy: the role of the nurse. *Nursing Times*, 90, 5–8.

Russell, A. (1996). Epilepsy. *Emergency Nurse*, 4, 9–15.

Taylor, M. P. (1996). *Managing Epilepsy in Primary Care*. Oxford: Blackwells.

Supracondylar fracture of the left humerus and consent

Ruth Sadik and Gill Campbell

Sian Williams, aged 7 years, was admitted to the ward following a fall from a swing in the local park. She walked into the Accident & Emergency department unaccompanied, crying and complaining of a great deal of pain in her left arm, which she was gingerly holding with her right hand. She was X-rayed, which confirmed a diagnosis of a supracondylar fracture of her left elbow. A collar and cuff were applied before receiving diclofenec 25 mg orally at 14:25 hours and she was transferred to the ward. On admission she had a temperature = 37.6°C, pulse = 112 beats min⁻¹ in her right arm and respiratory rate = 20 breaths min⁻¹. Her left radial pulse was present.

The police could not contact her parents and are currently trying to establish their whereabouts. Sian explains to the nursing staff that her father will be at work travelling around the area as a sales representative, while her mother will either be at home or in town, shopping. Sian understands that she has broken her arm and tells the nurse that her friend fell over last year breaking her leg, which she had to have put into plaster.

The staff nurse taking Sian's observations notes that her left radial pulse is becoming threadier and sends for the orthopaedic surgeon. A decision is made that surgery must proceed imminently if damage is not to occur to her left hand.

Question one: Discuss the legal considerations involved in taking Sian to theatre without her parents' explicit consent.

30 minutes

Question two: Using your knowledge of anatomy and physiology, explain the need for urgent surgery in Sian's case.

20 minutes

Question three: Rationalise the specific neurovascular observations Sian will require.

30 minutes

Question four: What factors will you need to consider while caring for Sian in the absence of her parents?

10 minutes

Time Allocation: **1 hour 30 minutes**

Answer to question one:
Discuss the legal considerations involved in taking Sian to theatre without her parents' explicit consent.

The rights of the child in relation to healthcare provision are subject to a variety of influences such as those of the parent or carer, other healthcare professionals, the culture, economics and government policies current at the time. As the child's advocate, especially in the absence of the parents, it is in the child's best interest if the nurse is intimately involved in discussing and/or gaining consent.

One of the most fundamental rights of the individual is to say what can and cannot be done to the person; the right to give or withhold consent (Fullbrook, 1998). The right for the mentally competent adult is firmly protected by law, which, if transgressed, can result in a civil case of trespass to the person, or a criminal case of assault and battery.

The Family Law Reform Act 1969, Section 8, states that a competent young person of 16 or 17 years can give consent to medical procedures without regard to parental wishes. However, this does not relate to withholding consent. This was legally tested in 1992 by child W, who wished to withhold consent for treatment and the law intervened (Dimond, 1996). While it may be seen as being in the child's best interests, it might also be seen as an attack on the right to autonomy and self determination.

Until recently, children < 16 years of age could not consent. Following the case of Gillick v Wisbech and Norfolk Health Authority (1986), the principle was put forward that children under this age could consent to treatment without parental authority if they were deemed to have the maturity and understanding to do so (Dimond, 1996). Gillick competence is an individual notion frequently delegated to junior medical staff to assess, who have minimal knowledge and experience in child development. In some cases this may lead to children waiting for surgery, who may, nonetheless be Gillick Competent. While some professionals involve children in decision-making about care, much communication rests on the premise that children need to be told what is being done, rather than consulted about whether it should be done.

Gillick Competent children may have consent given for them by their parent or guardian. However, like adults, consent need not be gained where there is an emergency situation and treatment urgently required (Elliott, 1998). The decision to adopt this approach rests with an individual's professional judgement.

Answer to question two:
Using your knowledge of anatomy and physiology explain the need for urgent surgery in Sian's case.

Supracondylar fracture of humerus is a common fracture in childhood and the distal fragment may be displaced posteriorly or anteriorly (Figure 17.1).

Sian's signs and symptoms suggest that the fracture is displaced; this is known as initial vascular embarrassment, or Volkmann's ischaemia, and it occurs in ~11% of cases (Schoenecker *et al.*, 1996). It occurs as muscle, blood vessels and nerves of the hand and arm are confined within inelastic boundaries (Ross, 1991), and known as compartments. The pressure inside these compartments may rise as a result of increasing oedema or haemorrhage.

Compression of the venous end of the capillary beds affects capillary bed emptying leading to a back-log and subsequent rise in hydrostatic pressure. The pressure forces fluid out of the capillaries into the surrounding tissues, thus further increasing compression of the brachial artery and radial nerve. The cyclical nature of this process rapidly leads to necrosis of the tissues.

This condition might be complicated by nerve injury. There is disagreement over the treatment of this type of fracture when the radial pulse is absent. However, the usual treatment is closed reduction (Garbuz *et al.*, 1996). Should closed reduction fail then open reduction, possibly using internal fixation should be attempted (Cheng *et al.*, 1995).

The failing radial pulse may be due to pressure or transection of the radial artery by the displaced bone or by swelling of the soft tissues. Nerve injuries are also common for the same reasons and occur in almost 60% of cases, the most common injury being a palsy of the anterior interosseous nerve (Garbuz *et al.*, 1996).

The nerve injuries will eventually recover, but may take up to one year.

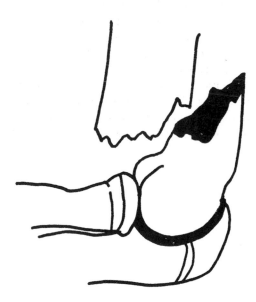

Figure 17.1. Anteriorly displaced supracondylar fracture of humerus.

Answer to question three:
Rationalise the specific neurovascular observations Sian will require.

The aim of Sian's care is to monitor her circulation and sensation using McRae's (1994) 5P classification (see Profile 10, Selina Robiero) to allow the early detection and remediation of compartment syndrome. The physiological mechanism of compartment syndrome is shown in Table 17.1.

Table 17.1. Compartment syndrome.

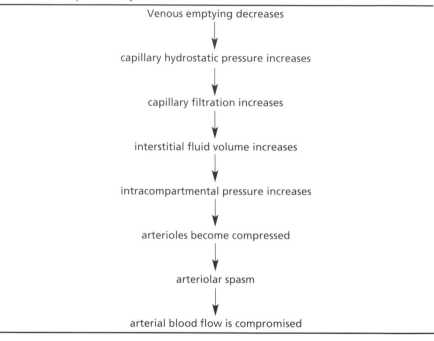

Venous emptying decreases

↓

capillary hydrostatic pressure increases

↓

capillary filtration increases

↓

interstitial fluid volume increases

↓

intracompartmental pressure increases

↓

arterioles become compressed

↓

arteriolar spasm

↓

arterial blood flow is compromised

Nursing assessment

To detect impairment of circulation the nurse will assess for:

- Pain: compression of the ulnar or radial nerve, in combination with the increased compartmental pressure, can lead to severe pain. However, this may also be an indicator of tissue hypoxia (Ross, 1991). Pain may not be relieved by opiates and may increase with elevation of the limb. The use of an appropriate pain assessment tool, such as Wong & Baker's (1988) faces scale (Wong *et al.*, 1999) (for more details on pain assessment, see Profile 23, Melanie Court) should be considered
- Movement: neurovascular assessment of the injured extremity may reveal weak active movement and some loss of sensation in the digits. As a result the nurse should test active extension, flexion, abduction and adduction of the fingers

- Sensation: nerve damage can occur at the time of injury or develop during the healing process. To test for sensation the nurse should use touch and pin prick to the skin and ask Sian to move the fingers of her right hand. Sian should also be monitored for complaints of tingling, burning, discomfort or altered sensation in general
- Circulation to the left arm: normally assessed by capillary refill time (see Profile 25, Caroline Davis). The colour and size of Sian's fingers on her left hand should be compared with those on her right to recognise that the circulation is not being compromised and an oedema occurring. Of great importance is the presence of the radial pulse, which should be recorded hourly (Wong *et al.*, 1999). The nurse should also check that Sian is not wearing any jewellery that could compromise the circulation. If she is, then – with her consent – it should be removed.

Answer to question four:
What factors will you need to consider while caring for Sian in the absence of her parents?

The following points should help you to care for Sian until her parents arrive:

- Assessment of needs should use a recognised framework. In the UK, the Activities of Living (Roper *et al.*, 1996) in conjunction with the Partnership Model (Casey, 1988) are frequently used to structure the assessment process
- Breathing: respiratory rate, depth and rhythm may indicate infection or disease process of which the anaesthetist should be informed
- Maintaining a safe environment: ability to understand and give consent to allow you to advocate for the child. Explain about pain assessment and analgesia (see Profile 23, Melanie Court)
- Communicating: sit close to Sian and at eye level. Put her at her ease and use age-appropriate language. Use open-ended questions and encourage discussion. To ascertain specific information, use focussed questions. Note Sian's non-verbal communication. Provide reassurance by acknowledging her concerns. Observe for signs of information overload. Allocate one nurse to take Sian through the peri-operative period
- Eating and drinking: to ensure safe anaesthetic induction ascertain the last time that Sian ate or drank. Explain about the need for nil orally from 2 h before the operation until after the operation. Ask whether she has any allergies or special needs with regard to implements. Weigh Sian to enable drugs to be accurately prescribed
- Eliminating: at age 7, Sian may occasionally be incontinent at night
- Personal cleansing and dressing: ensure that Sian is aware that she may have to wear a cotton gown and paper pants to theatre if her parents do not arrive with cotton garments in time. If her skin is dirty, Sian may need a bath or have an assisted full wash. Check her hair for nits and lice as theatre will need informing if she is infested (see Profile 10, Selina Robiero). Remove any nail varnish so that nail-bed perfusion can be monitored
- Controlling body temperature: record temperature to check for potential infection
- Mobilising: reassure Sian that she will be able to walk about when she has recovered from her operation. She will have a back-slab or full plaster in place, which she will have on for a number of weeks. She will need help with most activities of living initially
- Sleeping: explain that the anaesthetic sleep is different to usual sleep and that she will not be able to feel anything during the operation
- Dying: encourage Sian to air her concerns about dying under anaesthetic. Reassure her that she will wake up when the doctors tell her to, but not until the operation is completed

When Sian's family arrive the nurse should explain the injury sustained fully and the surgery required to correct it. They must also ascertain what input to everyday and nursing care the family want to contribute, if any.

Casey, A. (1988). A partnership with child and family. *Senior Nurse*, 18, 8–9.

Cheng, J. C., Lam, T. P., & Shen, W. J. (1995). Closed reduction and percutaneous prinning for Type III displaced supracondylar fractures of the humerus in children. *Journal of Orthopaedic Trauma*, 9, 511–515.

Dimond, B. (1996). *The Legal Aspects of Child Health Care*. London: Mosby.

Elliott, C. (1998). Consent and children. *Professional Nurse*, 13, 327–328.

Fullbrook, S. (1998). Medico-legal insights: consent and capacity: considerations for theatre nurses. *British Journal of Theatre Nursing*, 8, 31–33.

Garbuz, D. S., Leitch, K., & Wright, J. G. (1996). The treatment of supracondylar fractures in children with an absent radial pulse. *Journal of Pediatric Orthopaedics*, 16, 594–596.

McRae, R. (1994). *Practical Fracture Treatment*, 3rd edn. London: Churchill Livingstone.

Roper, N., Logan, W., & Tierney, A. (1996). *The Elements of Nursing*, 4th edn. London: Churchill Livingstone.

Ross, D. (1991). Acute compartment syndrome. *Orthopaedic Nursing*, 10, 33–38.

Schoenecker, P. L., Delgado, E., Rotman, M., Sicard, G., & Capoelli, A. (1996). Pulseless arm in association with totally displaced supracondylar fracture. *Journal of Orthopedic Trauma*, 10, 410–415.

Wong, D. L., Hockenberry-Eaton, M., Wilson, D., Winklestein, M. L., Ahmann, E., & DiVito-Thomas, P. A. (1999). *Whaley & Wong's Nursing Care of Infants and Children*, 6th edn. St Louis: Mosby.

Further reading

British Medical Association and The Law Society (1995). *Assessment of Mental Capacity: Guidance for Doctors and Lawyers*. London: BMA.

Fulton, Y. (1996). Children's rights and the role of the nurse. *Paediatric Nurse*, 8, 29–31.

Hendrick, J. (1997). *Legal Aspects of Child Health Care*. London: Chapman & Hall.

Web sites

(Accessed 22 June 2000).
[http://www.britishcouncil.org/governance/jusrig/lawact/childright/index.htm].

Bacterial endocarditis

Dawn Cowley and Sarah Standley

Stella Fielding is 7 years old. She is the eldest of the three children in her family and has a 6-week-old sister, Clarissa, and a 3-year-old brother, George. They live with their parents, Sam and Janine, in a four-bedroomed house, which is in the suburbs of a large city in the south of England. Shortly after birth, Stella was diagnosed with a small ventricular septal defect (VSD) that did not require surgical intervention.

Following a 3-week history of increasing fatigue, weakness, intermittent pyrexia and excessive sweating at night, Stella was seen by her local GP. Her mother reported that 4 weeks ago Stella had an extremely sore throat with difficulty swallowing, which was untreated and resolved within 7 days. She also noted that Stella had lost 2 kg in weight as her appetite had been very poor, which she had initially attributed to her sore throat. The weight loss and lack of appetite had continued after her throat had improved and Janine was concerned about her daughter. On examination, it was evident that a new tooth had recently erupted through the gums and the GP wondered if this could be the source of her recent problems. Stella was subsequently admitted to hospital where bacterial endocarditis was diagnosed.

Stella's mother cannot be resident on the ward as her husband is working away from home and she has Stella's siblings to care for. She can stay for short periods during the day when babysitters can be arranged.

Question one: Describe the endocardium of the heart.

5 minutes

Question two: What is bacterial endocarditis and who is at greatest risk of acquiring it?

10 minutes

Question three: Identify the clinical investigations Stella will require and her possible medical management.

20 minutes

Question four: Discuss the care Stella will require while she is on bed rest.

20 minutes

Question five: Outline the health education advice required by Stella and her family before discharge.

20 minutes

Time Allocation: **1 hour 15 minutes**

Answer to question one:
Describe the endocardium of the heart.

The endocardium is the smooth inner lining of the cavities of the heart and is continuous with the linings of the major blood vessels. It covers the valves of the heart and their associated tendons and facilitates a smooth flow of blood through the heart. The endocardium of the heart consists of squamous epithelial cells, minor blood vessels and bundles of smooth muscle (Wilson & Waugh, 1996; Mosby, 1998; Tortora & Grabowski, 2000).

Answer to question two:
What is bacterial endocarditis and who is at greatest risk of acquiring it?

Bacterial endocarditis is an infection of the endocardium that can also include the valves. Bacteria usually enters the blood stream via a localised site of infection in a high-risk individual. These sites of infection most commonly arise from oral lesions (including eruption of teeth), surgery, indwelling catheters or infective lesions of the integumentary system.

Bacteria become attached to scarred, damaged or malformed endothelium, which might include the valves. Clumps are formed from bacteria, fibrin and platelets and are known as vegetations (Davies, 1994; Mosby, 1998; Wong *et al.*, 1999).

Bacterial endocarditis occurs predominately in individuals with pre-existing anatomical abnormalities of the heart, those who have undergone cardiac surgery and individuals who have suffered cardiac damage due to disease process such as Kawasaki disease (an acute systemic febrile vasculitis) or rheumatic fever (Estlow, 1998).

Answer to question three:
Identify the clinical investigations Stella will require and her possible medical management.

To isolate the causative organisms blood cultures, throat swab, mouth swab and a urine sample will be obtained from Stella. Stella is known to have had a recent throat infection and it might be possible to obtain residual organisms. Stella has had a recently erupted tooth and this can be colonised by commensals, which might become pathogenic. Although she has no obvious signs of a urinary tract infection, this is a common site for infection in girls (Wong *et al.*, 1999). Sensitivity studies will identify the appropriate antibiotic treatment required.

An echocardiogram identifies possible cardiac abscesses and clumps of vegetation. An electrocardiogram (ECG) can identify congestive heart failure, dysrrhythmias and heart murmurs. Stella may have old ECGs from her infancy that can be used for comparison.

A chest X-ray will aid identification of cardiomegaly or pneumonia. Abdominal palpation will be performed by the doctors for signs of splenomegaly.

Medical management will comprise IV broad-spectrum antibiotics until negative blood cultures are obtained – not usually before 14 days. These are generally administered via a central venous catheter (Hickman line) to reduce problems associated with long-term administration of IV therapy (Davies, 1994; Wong *et al.*, 1999).

Answer to question four:
Discuss the care Stella will require while she is on bed rest.

The nurse's plan of care for Stella during the acute stage of her illness will need to give consideration to physical, psychological and social needs. Stella is likely to feel very scared and isolated. Preparation is required to help her understand the care she will need in these early stages of her illness. Many adults do not like the thought of blood tests and to a young child the idea could be terrifying (Manne *et al.*, 1993). Added to this are the various tests, medications and observations that she might have to face without the constant support and protection of her parents. The medical and nursing staff need to keep these thoughts uppermost in their care of Stella. Stella's parents should be encouraged to continue to care for their daughter to the level they feel able. They may also be scared, but with education, support and encouragement she will soon be able to participate fully in her care (Brennan, 1994).

Stella will be treated with IV antibiotics to destroy the bacteria. The medication will reach a therapeutic level within a few days. Administration of antipyretics and the monitoring of their effectiveness should allow the nurse to maintain Stella's TPR within normal limits for her age, temperature 36.5–37.3°C, pulse 75–115 beats min^{-1} and respirations 18–25 min^{-1} (Moules & Ramsey, 1998). In addition, it is important to consider environmental factors such as room temperature. Loose bedding and clothing could help to reduce her temperature; however, constant cuddling from relatives may increase her temperature. As the infection subsides, the TPR will return to normal.

Nausea and anorexia has been restricting Stella's diet and fluid intake. It is important to maintain fluid intake to at least her minimum requirement, which is calculated according to body weight (see Profile 25, Caroline Davis).

To aid assessment of Stella's level of hydration it is necessary to measure and document her fluid input and output. Other observations should include turgor of skin (Box 18.1), condition of mucous membranes – dry or moist, capillary refill time, TPR and urinalysis (Timby, 1996). These need monitoring and recording and any abnormality should be notified as appropriate.

Box 18.1. Assessment of skin turgor.

- Skin turgor: to measure this, the skin is pinched and lifted. In a healthy individual, when the skin is released it returns to its usual position immediately. When the patient is dehydrated, the skin takes longer to return. The more dehydrated the patient is the longer the skin will remain tented (Timby, 1996).

Nutritional and calorific intake is important for adequate growth and development; it is also important in maintaining tissue viability (Simpson, 1999). This is of particular concern as Stella requires a considerable amount of bed rest. On admission her weight should be obtained and recorded as this allows for comparison as well as being required for drug calculations. Weigh Stella on a biweekly basis and record. Abnormal weight increases can also be an early indicator of congestive cardiac failure. Involve Stella, the dietician and diet kitchen staff in food choices. Offering small portions will encourage her to eat. Document food eaten or left. Constipation is preventable for Stella by ensuring an adequate fluid intake and a diet containing soluble and insoluble non-starch polysaccharide (NSP) (Simpson, 1999). Offering popcorn, green vegetables, and fruit and vegetable with skins on will help to increase Stella's intake of NSP.

During the acute stage of her illness Stella will be required to stay on bed rest for at least 7 days. Immobility is an unnatural state and can be a causative factor in further problems, all of which are preventable with forethought and planning (Courtenay, 1999). Stella is at increased risk of thrombosis from bacterial vegetation becoming dislodged. Excessive movement might cause this vegetation to travel to any of the major organs forming blockages in small blood vessels. It is possible to prevent respiratory problems by ensuring Stella changes her position frequently. This allows normal drainage of secretions in the respiratory tract.

Through good pressure area care and observation one would expect to maintain the integrity of Stella's skin and prevent tissue breakdown, maintain vascular circulation and prevent a deep vein thrombosis. Ensure that Stella is washed and the bed linen and clothing is changed at least daily. Pressure area assessment and documentation should be performed at least twice daily. Stella and her parents should be educated about the risks and can be taught a physiotherapy regimen of exercise and movement in the form of play.

Stella will need considerable amounts of rest initially. She will need access to her personal belongings such as toys, books and audiotapes. Having familiar items around her will encourage a feeling of normality. It will be necessary to liaise with the school teacher, play therapist, family and friends. As advocated by Casey (1998), their involvement will facilitate development, reduce boredom, isolation and depression. These interventions should be of short duration, which can be increased as Stella's condition improves. Stella should then be nursed in the main ward area to allow her to socialise and to reduce her isolation.

Answer to question five:
Outline the health education advice required by Stella and her family before discharge.

Forward planning will allow Stella to return home with her family at the earliest possible time. Stella has a high risk of further episodes of bacterial endocarditis because of the VSD. To avoid a recurrence it is necessary to ensure her parents are educated in preventative measures (Giessel *et al.*, 2000). As Stella develops she will learn to take over the responsibility for her own health, so she should be included in this education programme to begin her learning process. Areas that may require attention are:

- Importance of good oral hygiene for Stella
- Prophylactic dose of antibiotics when having dental work; this may also be advocated until her dentition is complete
- Recognising the early signs and symptoms of bacterial infection and when to see her GP
- Although not currently important to Stella, Sam and Janine need information regarding the implications to Stella's health of pregnancy

This education should be informal. Give written information where possible to reinforce verbal and practical education. Follow each session with discussion, encouraging questions from Stella and her parents, to ascertain the development of their understanding and knowledge.

References

Brennan, A. (1994). Caring for children during procedures: a review of the literature. *Pediatric Nursing*, 20, 451–457.

Casey, A. (1998). A partnership with child and family. *Senior Nurse*, 18, 8–9.

Courtenay, M. (1999). Movement and mobility. In R. Hogston, & P. M. Simpson (eds), *Foundations of Nursing Practice* (216–239). Basingstoke: Macmillan.

Davies, P. (1994). Infective endocarditis. *Nursing Standard*, 8, 54–55.

Estlow, M. (1998). Prevention of infective endocarditis in the pediatric congenital heart population. *Pediatric Nursing*, 24, 17–21.

Giessel, B. E., Koenig, C. J., & Blake, R. L. (2000). Management of bacterial endocarditis. *American Family Physician*, 61, 1725–1732, 1739.

Manne, S., Bakeman, R., Jacobsen, P., & Redd, W. H. (1993). Children's coping during invasive medical procedures. *Behavior Therapy*, 24, 143–158.

Mosby's Medical Dictionary and Allied Health, 5th edn (1998). Mosby: London.

Moules, T., & Ramsay, J. (1998). *The Textbook of Children's Nursing*. Cheltenham: Stanley Thorns.

Simpson, P. M. (1999). Eating and drinking. In R. Hogston, & P. M. Simpson (eds), *Foundations of Nursing Practice* (93–132). Basingstoke: Macmillan.

Timby, B. K. (1996). *Fundamental Skills & Concepts in Patient Care*, 6th edn. Philadelphia: Lippincott.

Tortora, G. J., & Grabowski, S. R. (2000). *Principles of Anatomy and Physiology*, 9th edn. New York: Wiley.

Wilson, A., & Waugh, A. (1996). *Ross and Wilson's Anatomy and Physiology in Health and Illness*, 8th edn. London: Churchill Livingstone.

Wong, D. L., Hockenberry-Eaton, M., Wilson, D., Winkelstein, M. L., Ahmann, E., & DiVito-Thomas, P. A. (1999). *Whaley and Wong's Nursing care of infants and children*, 6th edn. St Louis: Mosby.

Further reading

Dajani, A. S., Taubert, K. A., Wilson, W., Bolger, A. F., Bayer, A., Ferrieri, P., Gewitz, M. H., Shulman, S. T., Nouri, S., Newburger, J. W., Hutto, C., Pallasch, T. J., Gage, T. W., Levison, M. E., Peter, G., & Zuccaro, G. (1997, accessed 24 July 2000). Prevention of bacterial endocarditis [http://www.americanheart.org/Scientific/statements/1997/079701.htm].

Payling, K. J. (1997). Kawasaki disease. *Professional Nurse*, 13, 108–109.

Peri-operative care for craniotomy

Christine Ward

Adam Frost is 10 years old and lives with his parents, Andy and Sandra. He has an older sister, Elizabeth, who is 14 years old. Despite the 4-year age gap, Adam and Elizabeth get on very well.

For some time, Adam has been experiencing headaches that seemed to get better as the day went on. He appeared to be unaffected by the headaches and continued to be his usual bubbly self. However, over the past 2 weeks Sandra noticed that Adam had been rather clumsy and often bumped into the furniture.

Sandra discussed the problem with Andy and they decide to make an appointment with the GP.

Following a neurological assessment the next day, the GP decided he would like to refer Adam to hospital for further investigations.

After being admitted by the nurse and doctor, a full neurological assessment was made. It was explained to Adam and his parents that the next stage was to have a CT (computed tomographic) scan of his head. The nurse explained that computers took these scans and that they gave a detailed picture of the brain. They were also completely painless.

The play specialist showed Adam some photographs of the scanner in preparation for this investigation.

After the scan, the doctor and nurse sat down with Andy and Sandra and explained that a lump, which might be a cyst or a tumour, had been found. It was advised that surgery was necessary to stop Adam's condition from deteriorating. After much discussion, Adam's parents agreed to the operation, which was scheduled for the next day. Sandra and Andy explained to Adam what was to happen and then the nurse and play specialist showed Adam more photographs in preparation for theatre and his return to the ward.

The next day Adam returned to the ward following a craniotomy and removal of a space-occupying lesion. Frozen section diagnosed a pilocytic astrocytoma.

Question one: Explain, using the pathophysiology of a pilocytic astrocytoma, the signs and symptoms that Adam has experienced.

20 minutes

Question two: Describe the peri-operative care that Adam will require for the first 48 h in hospital.

40 minutes

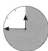

Time Allocation: **1 hour**

Answer to question one:
Explain, using the pathophysiology of a pilocytic astrocytoma, the signs and symptoms that Adam may experience.

A pilocytic astrocytoma is the second most common type of glioma in childhood. Most tumours are benign and are in the cerebellum (Rorke, 1999). The signs and symptoms are, therefore, initially related to the functions of the cerebellum, which are:

- Maintenance of balance and muscle tone
- Fine motor coordination

They tend to grow extensively in the subarachnoid space, a phenomenon not usually associated with a poor prognosis. Most are curable through surgical removal. However, recurrence and/or malignant transformation have been observed (Rorke, 1999). By the time the majority of tumours present with symptoms, they are large enough to present with the signs and symptoms of raised intracranial pressure (Box 19.1).

Box 19.1. Raised intracranial pressure.

- Seizure
- Personality disorder
- Headache
- Vomiting
- Unsteadiness
- Uncoordination of extremities
- Tremor
- Lapsing consciousness

Fortunately Adam's parents recognised symptoms early before the raised intracranial pressure led to a seizure. The other signs and symptoms will result from pressure on surrounding parts of the brain caused by the enlarging tumour.

Answer to question two:
Describe the peri-operative care that Adam will require for the first 48 h in hospital.

The initial pre-operative explanations given to Adam and his family by the nursing and play staff are vital in allaying fears. Douglas (1993) highlighted that parents who suffer anxiety are reluctant to inform their children about what is happening for fear of frightening them. This in turn deprives the child of the opportunity to learn how to cope with stress and fear appropriately. Sylva & Stein (1990) identified the importance of assessing the child and family before deciding on the level of information that would be most beneficial. They suggest that children who are out-going seek information, have some knowledge of hospital routines, are supported by their family and adapt better to potentially distressing information than more introverted children. Any kind of surgery on the brain is very emotive as it is one of the organs we know least about, and yet, conversely, it is well known that surgery to the brain is unpredictable and can result in potential long-term damage (Ater, 1998).

Before Adam can be expected to understand information about his condition and treatment, it is necessary to identify his level of understanding of how his body works (Douglas, 1993). Although Adam is 10 years old, research carried out by McEwing (1996) demonstrated that, even at 12 years old, many children could not make links between the function of one part of the body and others. This is essential for Adam, as he needs to understand that surgery on his brain can help in relieving problems with his balance, and may cause problems in the postoperative period that affect distant parts of his body.

It may also be appropriate to include Elizabeth in these explanatory sessions to evaluate and improve her knowledge of what is happening to Adam, and thus decrease her anxiety (Bossert, 1994; Holden, 1995).

Adam will also need preparing physically to ensure that he is well enough to withstand surgery and to gain information that will help the nursing and medical teams to plan and implement his care appropriately (Moules, 1998).

Adam's pre-operative care should include:

- Accurate weight (to ensure accurate drug dosage)
- Urine testing (to check for undiagnosed diabetes or renal damage)
- Discussion about pain control (to aid postoperative compliance)
- Informed consent for surgery (Adam and his parents have to be clear about the surgery and its outcomes)
- Fasting (2 h for fluid, 4 h for food are current recommendations) (Phillips *et al.*, 1994; Splinter, 1999)

Children of non-Caucasian ethnicity may require other tests such as blood for sickle cell or thalassaemia status, as the effects of anaesthesia can lead to a crisis (Moules, 1998).

To ensure Adam's safety during surgery the nurse should check that:

- He is wearing an identification bracelet(s) to ensure that the correct child receives the correct surgery

- Jewellery is removed if religion allows it or it is protected with tape (contact between metal jewellery and metal equipment can cause skin burns when diathermy is used
- Mucous membranes and nails should be in their natural state (lips and nail beds are used to assess perfusion during surgery)
- Note any loose teeth on Adam's pre-operative check list for they may become dislodged during intubation and block his airway
- Check that the consent form is signed and that all documentation and any skin marking are correct

At the allotted time Adam will be accompanied to theatre by a familiar member of the nursing team who will ensure that the transfer is carried out safely. Adam's parent(s) may also accompany him if it is their wish to help alleviate anxiety that Adam may experience about being anaesthetised. It is the responsibility of the accompanying nursing team member to look after the parent(s), and to ensure that they leave Adam when asked to by the anaesthetist.

Postoperatively, a qualified nurse will escort Adam back from the recovery area after s/he has ascertained the extent of surgery carried out, analgesic prescribed and that Adam's vital signs are stable and within normal limits.

Adam would return back to his bed area, which had been prepared with the necessary equipment needed to look after him postoperatively. This would include:

- Oxygen and suction
- IV infusion pump
- BP monitoring equipment
- Pulse oximetry equipment
- Pen torch
- Thermometer
- Up-dated guidelines or care plans
- Emergency trolley should be available in the event of a cardiac or respiratory arrest (Timby, 1996)

Adam would also have an IV infusion, which would be attached to a control pump to regulate the amount of fluid given. The fluid would be calculated according to Adam's weight. Assuming he weighed 30 kg, he would require 71 ml dextrose/saline hourly (see Profile 25, Caroline Davis).

Neurological observations would be carried out and recorded every 15–30 min for the first 6 h (see Profile 9, Jason King). It is important that these observations are carried out as it is in these first few hours that a haematoma or haemorrhage may occur, thus presenting as rising intracranial pressure.

Ater (1998) identified that emergencies occur quickly following craniotomy and the nurse's observations play a vital role in protecting the child's well-being. Any deterioration should be reported immediately (Wong *et al.*, 1999). If Adam's condition remains stable after 6 h, the observations may be recorded hourly, then 2 hourly as his condition allows.

Adam might have a small vacuum drain in place. The amount of drainage would be recorded frequently, for example hourly for the first 4 h, then 2–4 hourly until removed. Blood-stained fluid (25–75 ml) may be expected to drain in 24 h. He would also have a small dressing applied to his wound, which would be observed for any leakage and padded if necessary. If the dressing is soiled it should be reinforced with dry sterile gauze. The soiled area may be circled with a pen every hour. In this way continuous bleeding is easily recognised (Wong *et al.*, 1999).

Adam would be assessed for signs of pain (see Profile 21, John Reeves) and an analgesic would be given rectally with an anti-emetic. A side-effect of receiving an anaesthetic is vomiting so oral medication runs the risk of not being absorbed (Miller & Fioravanti, 1997).

The use of morphine is controversial with children who have had brain surgery as it can depress both respiratory effort and the level of consciousness. However, Wong *et al.* (1999) suggested that it can be given safely. Regardless of the type of analgesic administered, the intramuscular route should be avoided, as recent studies (Carter, 1994; Maikler, 1998; Boughton *et al.*, 1998) suggest that if pain relief is itself painful then it defeats its objective.

When Adam wishes, fluid and food may be given as tolerated, titrating the infusion as required.

To prevent pressure sores from developing, Adam would be turned every 2 h and encouraged to move around the bed as he is able. His hygiene and elimination needs would be met on demand, with the nursing team collaborating with Adam and his family.

Obviously, Adam's parents and sister would be very anxious and should be included in all aspects of his care to reassure themselves that he is alright. They should be informed of the outcome of surgery as soon as possible and given the opportunity to discuss any future implications.

References

Ater, J. (1998). Treatment of brain tumors in children: an overview. *Journal of Care Management*, 4, 96, 98, 100.

Bossert, E. (1994). Factors influencing the coping of hospitalized school-age children. *Journal of Pediatric Nursing: Nursing Care of Children and Families*, 9, 299–306.

Boughton, K., Blower, C., Chartrand, C., Dircks, P., Stone, T., Youwe, G., & Hagen, B. (1998). Impact of research on pediatric pain assessment outcomes. *Pediatric Nursing*, 24, 31–35.

Carter, B. (1994). *Child and Infant Pain.* London: Chapman & Hall.

Douglas, J. (1993). *Psychology and Nursing Children.* Basingstoke: Macmillan.

Holden, P. (1995). Psychosocial factors affecting a child's capacity to cope with surgery and recovery. *Seminars in Perioperative Nursing*, 4, 75–79.

Lewis, L. W., & Timby, B. K. (1998). *Fundamental Skills and Concepts in Patient Care.* London: Chapman & Hall.

Maikler, V. E. (1998). Pharmacologic pain management in children: a review of the literature. *Journal of Pediatric Nursing*, 13, 3–14.

McEwing, G. (1996). Children's understanding of their internal body parts. *British Journal of Nursing*, 15, 423–429.

Miller, S., & Fioravanti, J. (1997). *Pediatric Medications: A Handbook for Nurses.* London: Mosby.

Moules, T. (1998). Pre- and post-operative care. In T. Moules, & J. Ramsay (eds), *The Textbook of Children's Nursing* (378–385). Cheltenham: Stanley Thornes.

Phillips, S., Daborn, A. K., & Hatch, D. J. (1994). Pre-operative fasting for paediatric anaesthesia. *British Journal of Anaesthesia*, 73, 529–536.

Rorke, L. B. (1999). Pathology of brain and spinal cord tumors. In M. D. Choux, C. Rocco, A. D. Hockley, & M. L. Walker (eds), *Pediatric Neurosurgery* (395–426). New York: Churchill Livingstone.

Splinter, W. M. (1999). Pre-operative fasting in children. *Anesthesia and Analgesia*, 89, 80–89.

Sylva, K., & Stein, A. (1990). Effects of hospitalisation on young children. *Newsletter of Association for Child Psychology and Psychiatry*, 12, 3–9.

Timby, B. K. (1996) *Fundamental skills & concepts in patient care*, 6th edn. Philadelphia: Lippincott.

Wong, D. L., Hockenberry-Eaton, M., Wilson, D., Winkelstein, M. L., Ahmann, E., & DiVito Thomas, P. A. (1999). *Whaley and Wong's Nursing Care of Infants and Children*, 6th edn. St Louis: Mosby.

Further reading

Ainsworth, H. (1989). The nursing care of children undergoing craniotomy. *Nursing: Journal of Practice Education and Management*, 3, 5–8.

Allen, D. (1994). Paediatric coma scale. *Surgical Nurse*, 7, 14–16.

May, L., & Cater, B. (1995). *Child Health Care Nursing: Concepts, Theory and Practice*. Oxford: Blackwells.

Seeley, R. R., Stephens, T. D., & Tate, P. (1995). *Anatomy and Physiology*. London: Mosby.

Thompson, M. L. (1994). Information-seeking coping and anxiety in school-aged children anticipating surgery. *Children's Health Care*, 23, 87–97.

Pathophysiology of tonsils, post-tonsillectomy bleed, treatment and nursing care

Jane McConochie

Susan Latimer is 10 years old. Nine days ago she was in hospital having had her adenoids and tonsils removed.

Since her discharge from hospital she was well for the first few days but her throat remained very sore. She found eating and drinking very difficult even though she was taking paracetamol and ibuprofen regularly. Susan's mother had tried very hard to get her to eat and drink but found it hard, and most of the time was unsuccessful, although small amounts of fluid were taken on occasions.

On waking this morning, Susan's throat was particularly sore and she feels nauseated. Analgesics have had little effect and her nausea persists.

During the morning she is very sick bringing up fresh blood, clots and stale blood. Her mother takes her temperature, which is 38°C. Susan continues to bring up small amounts of fresh blood and her worried mother contacts the GP. He visits Susan at home and following his examination advises that admission to hospital is necessary.

On arrival in the children's ward a nurse assesses Susan. She is quiet and withdrawn, her temperature is now 38.5°C, her pulse = 120 beats min⁻¹ and respirations = 22 breaths min⁻¹. There is no excessive swallowing, but every now and then she spits out a small amount of fresh blood and saliva.

Following examination, the doctor feels that at present there is no need to take Susan to theatre. He explains to Susan and her mother that the tonsil bed shows signs of infection and that there is a small bleeding point apparent. Having prescribed the appropriate treatment he says that he will review her later that day.

Question one: Outline the pathophysiology of the tonsils and adenoids.

10 minutes

Question two: Describe the types of bleeding/haemorrhage that can occur following a tonsillectomy.

10 minutes

Question three: Describe the management and nursing care that Susan may need during the first 24 h following her admission.

20 minutes

Time Allocation: **40 minutes**

Answer to question one:
Outline the pathophysiology of the tonsils and adenoids.

The tonsils and adenoids are composed of lymphatic nodules that form a ring at the junction of the naso- and oro-pharynx (Tortora & Grabowski, 2000). The tonsils protect the gastrointestinal system from infection. As one swallows, the tonsils are compressed ejecting leucocytes into the food, which kill the bacteria before they get into the stomach. Cilia in the nose collect debris and bacteria when air is breathed through the nose; this may be infected, and the adenoids protect the respiratory tract from this infection (Figure 20.1).

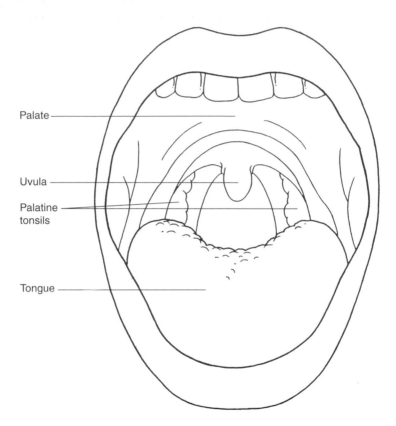

Palate

Uvula

Palatine tonsils

Tongue

Figure 20.1. Position of the palatine tonsils.

Answer to question two:
Describe the types of bleeding/haemorrhage that can occur following a tonsillectomy.

There are three types of haemorrhage that can occur as a complication of tonsillectomy (Chambers, 1999):

- Primary haemorrhage which occurs during surgery
- Intermediary (reactionary) haemorrhage, which occurs within 24 h of surgery as a result of BP stabilisation (Colman, 1992; Chambers, 1999)
- Secondary haemorrhage, which may occur some time between the fifth and tenth day post-surgery due to infection in the tonsillar fossae (Colman, 1992)

Answer to question three:
Describe the management and nursing care that Susan may need during the first 24 h following her admission.

Susan's care is structured on Roper *et al.*'s (1996) activities of living model:

- Mobility: Susan will be advised to rest, getting up only to go to the toilet with assistance. Loss of blood volume can lower BP and cause fainting
- Eating and drinking: IV fluids will be started (for details on care of an IV infusion, see Profile 25, Caroline Davis). Haemoglobin levels will be checked, and if Susan is anaemic a blood transfusion will be given. Once Susan's nausea and vomiting stops, diet and fluids will be introduced. An accurate fluid balance chart will be kept. While Susan is nil by mouth it is important that she receives regular oral hygiene and is given the opportunity to brush her teeth. If brushing alone is insufficient to remove hardened blood/debris then sodium bicarbonate can be tried. This is diluted 1 part sodium bicarbonate to 160 parts water (one teaspoon in one tumbler) and it is important to remember that it is not pleasant to taste (HEA, 1997)
- Body temperature: temperature, pulse and respiration will be monitored and recorded 4 hourly. Increases in these values may indicate infection. The doctor should prescribe IV antibiotics. BP is not generally monitored as in children < 8 years of age it tends to be labile (DeSwiet *et al.*, 1992) and is an unreliable indicator of impending shock. However, as Susan is 10 years old her BP should be recorded with her other vital signs
- Safety: 6% hydrogen peroxide gargles may be prescribed. If the solution is not premixed then 15 ml should be added to half a tumbler of cold water (HEA, 1997). This helps clean debris from the tonsillar fossae. Analgesics will be prescribed and given as necessary
- Communication: Susan and her mother will need reassurance and a full explanation of all necessary treatments

If the bleeding does not stop then Susan might need to be taken to theatre for examination under anaesthetic and ligation of a bleeding vessel. Susan will be allowed home once she is eating and drinking and has remained apyrexial for 24 h.

References

Chambers, N. (1999). *Wound Management*. In R. Hogston, & P. Simpson (eds), *Foundations of Nursing Practice* (240–266). Basingstoke: Macmillan.

Colman, B. (1992). *Diseases of the Nose Throat and Ear and Head and Neck*, 14th edn. London: Churchill Livingstone.

DeSwiet, M., Fayers, P., & Shinebourne, E. (1992). Blood pressure in the first ten years of life. The Brompton Study. *British Medical Journal*, 304, 23–26.

Health Education Authority (1997). *The Scientific Basis of Dental Health Education*. London: HEA.

Roper, N., Logan, W. W., & Tierney, A. J. (1996). *The Elements of Nursing*, 4th edn. Edinburgh: Churchill Livingstone.

Tortora, G., & Grabowski, S. (2000). *Principles of Anatomy and Physiology*, 9th edn. New York: Wiley.

Further reading

Anon. (n.d., accessed 24 July 2000). Tonsils and adenoids [http://www.ent-surgeon.co.uk/tonsil_&_adenoids.htm].

Bandolier (n.d., accessed 24 July 2000). Tonsillectomy for sore throats [http://www.jr2.ox.ac.uk/bandolier/band55/b55-4.htm].

Slipped upper femoral epiphysis, similar orthopaedic conditions and complications of bed rest

Jane McConochie

John Reeves is 10 years old and has been admitted to the ward from A&E with a slipped upper femoral epiphysis of his left hip.

He has been experiencing pain in his left hip for ~3 months. At first, the pain was only felt occasionally, but as the weeks went by the pain became more intense, causing him to limp badly and preventing him from participating in sporting activities at school.

Mrs Reeves had taken John to the GP on several occasions where he was prescribed painkillers and told that it was possibly growing pains.

John's hip pain became more severe than usual and he was finding it almost impossible to walk, so Mrs Reeves decided that she would attend A&E rather than see her GP again. Following a series of hip X-rays a diagnosis of slipped upper femoral epiphysis was made.

On admission to the ward John was a pleasant but very anxious boy. This was his first admission to hospital and he was worried about having difficulty walking. Once he was resting in bed the pain eased and his left leg tended to rotate externally.

Having been examined by the doctor it was explained to John and his mother that the growing plate on John's thigh bone has slipped downwards and backwards (Figure 21.1).

It is explained to them that John will require an operation to pin the slipped epiphysis back into position to prevent the condition from getting any worse. The operation needs to be carried out within the next 24 h, and until then John is to remain resting on his bed.

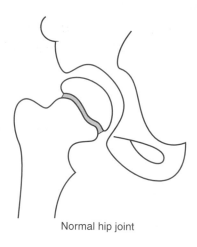

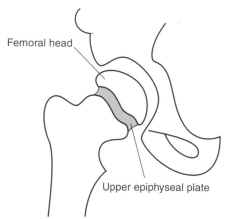

Femoral head

Upper epiphyseal plate

Slipped upper femoral epiphysis

Figure 21.1. Normal hip and slipped upper femoral epiphysis.

Question one: Describe the range of orthopaedic conditions that can present with pain in the hip and/or knee and refusal or reluctance to walk.

15 minutes

Question two: Postoperatively, what interventions could be used to assess and control John's pain?

15 minutes

Question three: Outline the complications of bed rest.

15 minutes

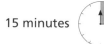

Time Allocation: **45 minutes**

Answer to question one:

Describe the range of orthopaedic conditions that can present with pain in the hip and/or knee and refusal or reluctance to walk.

Condition and causes are:

- Slipped upper femoral epiphysis: hormonal imbalance; over-weight
- Perthes' disease: reduced blood to the head of the femur
- Septic arthritis: infection in a joint
- Irritable hip (transient synovitis): cause unknown
- Osteomyelitis: infection in a bone
- Developmental dysplasia of the hip: hormonal imbalance; breech presentation; twinning and large infant size
- Juvenile chronic arthritis: inflammation of joints; growth plates may fuse prematurely

Answer to question two:
Postoperatively, what intervention could be used to assess and control John's pain?

McCaffery & Beebe (1989: 13) defined pain as being 'whatever the experiencing person says it is, existing whenever the person says it does'. This implies that the underlying philosophy towards the child in pain is one of being believed. Baker & Wong (1987) introduced a valuable nemonic for the principles of assessing pain in children:

- Question the child
- Use a pain rating scale
- Evaluate behaviour and physiologic changes
- Secure parental involvement
- Take the cause of pain into account
- Take action and evaluate results

which can be usefully employed with John and his family.

There are tools available to help the nursing staff to identify John's pain level and to help him achieve effective pain management. However, it must be remembered that elimination of all pain is not always achievable (Carter and Dearmun, 1995), and the nurse should aim to relieve as much as is possible.

As John is 10 years old, the most appropriate tools are:

- Word-Graphic Rating Scale (Testler *et al.*, 1991)
- Visual Analogue Scale (Devine, 1990)

These respect John's developmental abilities with regard to numeracy, while acknowledging that he may regress through the pain experience to a level where he is more comfortable with visual recognition.

Interventions for use with the child in pain include both pharmacological and non-pharmacological methods.

Pharmacological interventions

The following analgesics may be used as pain relief:

- Opioides, e.g. morphine, pethidine, dihydrocodeine
- Co-proxamol
- Co-dydramol
- Diclofenac
- Paracetamol

This medication may be given as follows:

- IV: using this route, the opiates can be given as a bolus, an infusion or as patient controlled analgesics (PCA)
- Intramuscularly (IM): opiates and diclofenac can be given by this route
- Rectally (PR): paracetamol and diclofenac may be given as suppositories
- Orally (PO): all the listed medication can be given by this route

The choice of route should be discussed with John and his mother. However, consideration should be given to the severity of the pain, time taken for the route to be effective, availability of drug to be administered via the desired route, and age and compliance of the child (Niederhauser, 1997). Before surgery it could be explained to John that postoperatively giving him analgesics as an IV infusion or PCA could control his pain. As he gets better, this method of pain control could be withdrawn and oral analgesics introduced. Non-pharmacological methods of pain relief can be used alongside analgesic drugs at all times.

For further information on drug administration and pain control, see Profile 23 (Melanie Court).

Non-pharmacological methods

Non-pharmacological methods of controlling John's pain may involve:

- Diversional play including creativity and drama
- Massage
- Aromatherapy
- Reflexology
- Acupressure
- Shiatsu

The nurse not qualified to administer some of the more specialised therapies may wish to employ the simpler techniques. These are diversional play and those involving touch such as stroking or gentle rubbing (Carter and Dearmun, 1995). The golden rule for any nurse is to ensure that informed consent is gained and that no harm befalls the patient (*Nursing Times*, 1994).

Answer to question three:
Outline the complications of bed rest.

Immobility imposed on John through bed rest can lead to physiologic and psychological complications (Health, 1995). According to Styrcula (1994), these are:

- Nutritional: loss of appetite can lead to poor diet and this can progress to skin breakdown and delayed wound healing
- Elimination: constipation and urinary tract infections might occur through poor food and fluid intake. Bone demineralisation may result in renal calculi
- Respiratory: poor posture and shallow breathing can increase the risk of chest infections
- Skin care: lack of movement and poor nutrition can lead to skin breakdown
- Cardiovascular: venous stasis may occur which may cause oedema and/or a deep vein thrombosis
- Psychosocial: boredom, alterations in sleep patterns and behavioural changes may occur
- Movement and mobility: joint stiffness, muscle wastage and contractures

References

Baker, C., & Wong, D. (1987). QUESTT: a process of pain assessment in children. *Orthopaedic Nursing*, 6, 11.

Carter, B., & Dearmun, A. K. (eds) (1995). *Child Health Care Nursing*. Oxford: Blackwells.

Devine, T. (1990). Pain management in paediatric oncology. *Paediatric Nursing*, 2, 10–13.

Health, H. B. M. (ed.) (1995). *Foundation in Nursing Theory and Practice*. London: Times Mirror International.

McCaffery, M., & Beebe, A. (1989). *Pain: A Clinical Manual for Nursing Practice*. St Louis: Mosby.

Niederhauser, V. P. (1997). Prescribing for children: issues in pediatric pharmacology. *Nurse Practitioner*, 22, 16–30.

Nursing Times (1994). *Nursing Times Guide to Using Complementary Therapies in Nursing*. London: Nursing Times.

Styrcula, L. (1994). Traction basics: Part IV. Traction for lower extremities. *Orthopaedic Nursing*, 13, 59–68.

Testler, M., Savedra, M., Holzemer, W., Wilkie, D., Ward, J., & Paul, S. (1991). The word-graphic rating scale as a measure of childrens' and adolescents' pain intensity. *Research in Nursing and Health*, 14, 361–371.

Further reading

Francis, S., & Ridge, K. (1993). Aspects of drug therapy for pediatric surgical patients. *Hospital Pharmacy Practice*, 3, 313–322.

Kanneh, A. (1998). Pharmacological principles applied to children. *Paediatric Nursing*, 10, 17–20.

Sanderson, H., & Carter, A. (1994). Healing hands. *Nursing Times*, 90, 46–49.

Waterlow, J. (1997). Pressure sore risk assessment in children. *Paediatric Nursing*, 9, 21–24.

Wink, D. M. (1991). Giving infants and children drugs. *Maternal and Child Nursing*, 16, 317–321.

Surgical causes of abdominal pain, and postoperative nursing care

Jane McConochie

Sally Whittaker, aged 13 years, was admitted to the ward with abdominal pain, having been sent to hospital by her GP. She had started complaining of abdominal pain the previous evening and since that time the pain had become progressively worse.

When examined by her GP he found that she was tender when touched in the central abdomen but particularly in the right iliac fossa and that there was some guarding with rebound. Her temperature was 37.6°C, pulse = 90 beats min^{-1} and respiratory rate = 16 min^{-1}. She had loss of appetite, but no vomiting and her last normal bowel movement was the previous morning.

The GP suggested a possible diagnosis of appendicitis and that she needed immediate admission to hospital. The GP's findings were recorded in the letter Sally and her mother took with them on admission to the ward.

On admission Sally looked pale and drawn. She finds it uncomfortable to walk and is only too grateful to be shown to a cubicle and to lie down on the bed with her knees bent. The nurse repeated her temperature, which remains at 37.6°C and explains to Sally that a midstream specimen of urine is required. Sally is given instructions on how the urine sample is to be collected. On ward testing the urine shows nothing abnormal. Local anaesthetic is applied to the back of her hand and antecubital fossa before a blood test is taken. Sally is told to remain nil by mouth.

The doctor examines Sally who, apart from an upper respiratory tract infection 2 weeks ago, is normally fit and well. The findings are similar to those of the GP. Blood is taken for full blood count, and urea and electrolytes. An IV infusion is commenced to maintain Sally's hydration. The doctor says he will review her later when the blood results are known. An hour later the results show that they are within normal limits except that the white cell count is 17.5×10^9 cells l^{-1} (normal 4.5–13.5×10^9 cells l^{-1}).

On receiving the results, the doctor decides that Sally should go to theatre for an appendicectomy.

Question one: List the conditions that may cause abdominal pain in children.

20 minutes

Question two: Discuss the postoperative care that Sally may require during the first 24 h following surgery.

30 minutes

Time Allocation: **50 minutes**

Answer to question one:
List the conditions that may cause abdominal pain in children.

The conditions causing abdominal pain in children are many, which makes diagnosis very difficult, and they include:

- Throat infections
- Mesenteric adenitis
- Chest infections
- Appendicitis
- Meckel's diverticulum
- Irritable bowel syndrome
- Intestinal obstruction
- Colitis
- Crohn's disease
- Urinary tract infection
- Renal calculi
- Ovarian cyst
- Adhesions following abdominal surgery
- Coeliac disease (gluten-sensitive enteropathy)
- Diabetes mellitus
- Henöch–Schölein purpura

In throat infections and mesenteric adenitis the copious mucous secretions that accompany upper respiratory tract infections lead to an increase in the pH of the stomach. Subsequently, ingested bacteria are less likely to be destroyed by the gastric acid. This allows bacteria to enter the small intestine and to gain access to the lymphatic system leading to mesenteric adenitis.

Chest infections cause splinting of the diaphragm and abdominal muscles leading to abdominal pain. Inflammation of the small or large bowel, which may be found in Meckel's diverticulum, irritable bowel syndrome, colitis and Crohn's disease will be accompanied by changes in patterns of defaecation which is usually diarrhoea.

In coeliac disease the damaged wall of the small intestine along with anorexia will cause abdominal pain. Inflammation of structures within the abdominal or pelvic cavities such as the ovaries, bladder or peritoneum may cause abdominal pain by stimulation of the vagus nerve.

Henöch–Schölein purpura leads to abdominal pain through small infarctions in the small intestine.

For further information regarding these conditions, see Further reading.

Answer to question two:
Discuss the postoperative care that Sally may require during the first 24 h following surgery.

Sally's bed area will be prepared, ensuring that oxygen and suction are available and working. This equipment is vitally important in case Sally's airway was to become obstructed. The nurse will collect Sally, with her parents, from the recovery room. Before leaving the recovery room the ward nurse must assure herself that she understands the procedure that Sally has undergone and that Sally can maintain her own airway. This can be established by checking that Sally has a cough reflex and responds to her name. The nurse must also ensure that all medication and fluids that may be required in the immediate postoperative period have been prescribed (Timby, 1996).

On return to the ward the nurse will monitor and record Sally's temperature, pulse, respirations and wound status. These observations will require monitoring half hourly, then hourly and eventually 4 hourly as her condition stabilises. This monitoring is to detect potential complications such as haemorrhage or hypovolaemic shock, which can be identified by a rising pulse and a falling BP, or infection, identified by a rising temperature, pulse and respiration rate. Table 22.1 identifies the possible causes for changes in the vital signs.

Table 22.1. Vital signs and possible causes (Wong *et al.*, 1999).

Vital sign	Possible cause
Tachycardia	hypovolaemic shock pyrexia pain early respiratory distress drugs, e.g. atropine
Bradycardia	decreased oxygenation stimulation of the vagus nerve raised intracranial pressure late respiratory distress drugs
Increased respiratory rate	respiratory distress hypervolaemia pyrexia pain
Decreased respiratory rate	anaesthetics/opiates pain
Hypertension	hypervolaemia raised intracranial pressure high $PaCO_2$ drugs
Hypotension	drugs shock
Pyrexia	infection external factors malignant hyperpyrexia
Hyperthermia	drugs external factors cold intravenous fluids

Peritonitis is a major risk following surgery, and the main sites for abscess formation are subdiaphragmatic, hepatic and retroperitoneal. This is one of the primary reasons for sitting Sally upright, well supported by pillows during the postoperative period.

Sally's input and output should be monitored and recorded accurately, including IV fluids. Lack of bowel sounds or flatus or abdominal distension could indicate a paralytic ileus and oral fluids and diet should not be introduced until either bowel sounds have returned or flatus is passed. If Sally says she feels hungry, this is often a sign that the bowel is functioning again.

Following assessment of Sally's pain level (see Profiles 21, John Reeves, and 23, Melanie Court), ensure that analgesics are given to keep Sally comfortable. This will allow her to move more freely, thus decreasing the likelihood of post-operative complications arising (Carter & Dearmun, 1995) such as the formation of pressure sores (see Profile 8, Samantha Lawrence).

If Sally is prescribed antibiotics, the nurse must ensure that they are given by the correct route and at the appropriate times.

Personal cleansing is important. During the first 24 h post-surgery a bed bath would be advisable, and Sally should be consulted about whether she would like her mother to help. Sally's mother should feel confident to do this. As Sally will be taking nothing by mouth, ensure that oral hygiene is carried out at least three times daily (Campbell & Glasper, 1995).

Support of Sally's parents will include keeping them informed of any treatments that she may need, reassurance to ensure reduction of anxiety and communicating to all in language and media that they will understand.

References

Campbell, S., & Glasper, E. A. (eds) (1995). *Whaley and Wong's Children's Nursing*. London: Mosby.

Carter, B., & Dearmun, A. K. (eds) (1995). *Child Health Care Nursing*. Oxford: Blackwells.

Timby, B. K. (1996). *Fundamental Skills and Concepts in Patient Care*, 6th edn. Philadelphia: Lippincott.

Wong, D. L., Hockenberry-Eaton, M., Winkelstein, M. L., Wilson, D., Ahmann, E., & DiVito-Thomas, P. A. (1999). *Whaley & Wong's Nursing Care of Infants and Children*, 6th edn. St Louis: Mosby.

Further reading

Anon. (1992). Ulcerative colitis [http://pharminfo.com/pubs/msb/nih_ibd.htm].

Anon. (n.d., accessed 1 August 2000). Differential diagnosis: Crohn's disease [http://www.lunis.luc.edu/radiology/Appendicitis/crohn1.htm].

Anon. (n.d., accessed 1 August 2000). Differential diagnosis: mesenteric adenitis [http://www.lunis.luc.edu/radiology/Appendicitis/mesenter.htm].

Anon. (n.d., accessed 1 August 2000). Diverticular disease of the small bowel [http://www.merck.com/pubs/mmanual/section3/chapter33/33e.htm].

Anon. (n.d., accessed 1 August 2000). Guidelines for the management of patients with coeliac disease [http://www.bsg.org.uk/guidelines/27722.htm].

Anon. (n.d., accessed 1 August 2000). Henoch–Schölein purpura [http://www.mc.vanderbilt.edu/peds/pidl/nephro/henoch.htm].

Anon. (n.d., accessed 1 August 2000). Meckel's diverticulum [http://www.mc.vanderbilt.edu/peds/pidl/gi/meckel.htm].

Anon. (n.d., accessed 1 August 2000). Module 2 – Diseases and malfunctions: minicourse 4 – the acute abdomen [http://www4.ncsu.edu/eos/users/w/wes/homepage/SIMS/Module2/GE2_4.htm].

Anon. (n.d., accessed 1 August 2000). Ovarian cysts [http://www.ppphealthcare.co.uk/html/health/ovarcyst.htm].

Bisset, A. F. (1998). The case for clinical audit of emergency readmissions after appendicectomy [http://www.rcsed.ac.uk/journal/old/4340012.htm].

Kubba, A. K., Price, R. F., Smith, G., & Palmer, R. (1998). Appendicectomy and ulcerative colitis [http://www.rcsed.ac.uk/journal/old/4340007.htm].

Vade, A., Salomon, C. G., Kalbhen, C. L., & Halama, J. R. (n.d., accessed 1 August 2000). Clinical and diagnostic imaging correlates in appendicitis in children: a computer aided teaching program [http://www.lunis.luc.edu/radiology/Appendicitis/default.htm].

Abdominal injury, pain and peri-operative care

Ruth Sadik and Gill Campbell

Melanie is a 13-year-old kicked by her horse when she went to feed him before leaving for school. When she had not returned home by 08:00 hours her mother went looking for her and she found her daughter dazed and winded, lying against the wall of the stable. An ambulance was called and Melanie was taken to the hospital where she was admitted to the children's ward.

Three hours following admission, Melanie vomited 250 ml bile-stained fluid. Her rising pulse and falling BP are beginning to indicate that she is bleeding somewhere and doctors suspect a ruptured liver as she has some tenderness and guarding in the right upper quadrant of her abdomen. Her mother is visibly shaken by the seriousness of the doctors provisional diagnosis and requests that her husband is summoned home from his posting with the Royal Navy in Gibraltar as she has no one else to care for Alistair, aged 9, and 11-year-old Amy.

As Melanie continues to vomit, a nasogastric tube is passed and she has 220 ml bile-stained fluid in her stomach. Melanie weighs 45 kg, so an IV infusion of dextrose saline is commenced at 105 ml h^{-1} (for details on calculation of fluid requirements, see Profile 25, Caroline Davis). The surgeons decide to evaluate the effect of fluid replacement on Melanie's condition, but within an hour she deteriorates. Her vital signs are pulse rate = 112 beats min^{-1}, respiration rate = 24 breaths min^{-1}, BP = 90/50 mmHg, and she is pale and clammy. It is decided that she will be taken to theatre for a laparotomy. Following a resection of a damaged liver lobe, she is transferred from theatre to the intensive care unit (ICU).

Question one: What specific nursing care will Melanie require during her peri-operative period?

30 minutes

Question two: List how you would recognise that Melanie was in pain.

15 minutes

Time Allocation: **45 minutes**

Answer to question one:
What specific nursing care will Melanie require during her peri-operative period?

The principles of care throughout this period will revolve around Melanie's airway, pulse rate, BP, respiration, abdominal girth, control of pain and fluid intake and output.

Observations of Melanie's airway will be the first priority. She will be breathing spontaneously before surgery and possibly on her return from theatre to ICU. Care must be taken to ensure that her airway does not become obstructed, particularly with vomit. Aspirating her nasogastric tube or leaving it on free drainage will help alleviate this, but a suction apparatus should be at hand. If Melanie is still intubated, then regular application of suction and support of the endotracheal tube should ensure its patency.

Melanie's respiratory rate and pattern will be continuously monitored. A respiratory rate of 12–16 breaths min⁻¹ (Hazinski, 1999) should be seen. A slower rate could be associated with opiate usage. Melanie will require pain relief throughout this period, but is covered below. The nurse must monitor the effectiveness of the analgesic given as well as its potential side-effects (Wong *et al.*, 1999). A faster respiratory rate could indicate anxiety and pain. The nurse can help reduce or alleviate anxiety by informing Melanie about what is happening and allowing her parents to stay with her if she wishes (Hogg, 1994; Jones, 1995). The nurse should understand that the depth of breathing can be affected by 'splinting' of the diaphragm which can occur as a result of a build up of air in the stomach, pain or from internal bleeding leading to a 'tense' abdomen.

Oxygen therapy may be administered and its effectiveness gauged by pulse oximetry. Cardiovascular monitoring will include heart rate and rhythm, BP, temperature and capillary refill time (CRT) (see Profile 25, Caroline Davis). These readings can be compared with Melanie's pre-operative observations so that a trend can be established. If the trend goes up and Melanie becomes hypertensive and tachycardic, this could be indicative of anxiety and pain. Alternatively, hypotension and tachycardia could indicate haemorrhage or hypovolaemia, as the heart beats faster to try to maintain cardiac output with a reduced circulating volume. This could also be accompanied by a prolonged CRT, a distended abdomen and a lowered peripheral temperature as a result of vasoconstriction to preserve circulation to the vital organs.

To assess any distension of Melanie's abdomen, girth measurements should be carried out regularly. It is important the measurement is taken with Melanie lying supine and the tape measure in the same place (this may require marking the skin so that the same point can be measured to ensure accuracy). A paper tape measure should be used for accuracy but the nurse should be aware of the danger of paper cuts to Melanie's skin.

Postoperatively Melanie will have abdominal drains *in situ* and the nurse must observe and record the amount and type of drainage. Blockage of the drains may result in abdominal distension. Large quantities of fresh blood indicate a bleeding point and this must be acted on.

As Melanie will be 'nil by mouth' during this period she will require hydration via an IV infusion as commenced pre-operatively (for care of an IV infusion, see Profile 25, Caroline Davies). Fluid lost via the nasogastric tube may also need to be substituted IV.

Melanie will probably be catheterised postoperatively but throughout the period her urinary output must be measured and recorded.

Usual peri-operative care will be implemented in conjunction with this specific care.

Answer to question two:
List how you would recognise that Melanie was in pain.

Melanie states the site and nature of the pain (client description is the most important factor in pain assessment; Wong *et al.*, 1999):

- Behaviour: might appear withdrawn or aggressive
- Tachypnoea/reluctance to deep breathe
- 'Guarding' of the painful area
- Tachycardia: due to activation of the adrenergic nervous system
- Hypertension: due to activation of the adrenergic nervous system
- Pupil dilation: due to activation of the adrenergic nervous system
- Position in bed: Melanie may be sat rigidly in one position to minimise her pain

A useful tool for assessing Melanie's pain would be QUESTT, as developed by Baker & Wong (1987) (see Profile 21, John Reeves), in collaboration with a pictorial scale such as the Wong & Baker (1988) faces scale, as they found it favourable to children from 3 to 18 years of age. Gaining Melanie's cooperation in assessing her pain can give her a sense of control, which in turn can result in decreasing pain perception (Moules and Ramsay, 1998).

References

Baker, C., & Wong, D. (1987). QUESTT: a process of pain assessment in children. *Orthopaedic Nurse*, 6, 11–21.

Hazinski, F. M. (1999). *Care of the Critically Ill Child*. St Louis: Mosby.

Jones, S. (1995). The development of the pediatric nurse specialist. *British Journal of Nursing*, 4, 34–36.

Hogg, K. (1994). Don't let cure be at the expense of care. *Professional Nurse*, 9, 655–656, 668–670.

Moules, T., & Ramsay, J. (1998). *The Textbook of Children's Nursing*. Cheltenham: Stanley Thornes.

Wong, D., & Baker. C. (1988). Pain in children: comparison of assessment scales. *Pediatric Nursing*, 14, 9–17.

Wong, D. L., Hockenberry-Eaton, M., Winkelstein, M. L., Wilson, D., Ahmann, E., & DiVito-Thomas, P. A. (1999). *Whaley & Wong's Nursing Care of Infants and Children*, 6th edn. St Louis: Mosby.

Further reading

Hirsch, M. P., & McKenna, C. J. (1996). Abdominal pain in children: surgical considerations. *Topics in Emergency Medicine*, 18, 49–61.

O'Conner-Von, S. (n.d., accessed 1 August 2000). Pediatric pain assessment [http://coninfo.nursing.uiowa.edu/sites/PedsPain/Assess/Chiasst.htm].

Scheb, D., & Pasero, C. (n.d., accessed 1 August 2000). Basic pain assessment in adults [http//www.baxter.com/doctors/iv_therapy_CE/Basic_Pain/painadult.htm].

Sickle cell anaemia

Wendy Jones

Gemma Daniels, a 14-year-old girl, is of West African descent. She is homozygous for sickle cell anaemia, being diagnosed after her first crisis at 8 months of age. She lives with her parents and three younger brothers on an estate some miles from the hospital. Two of her brothers have sickle cell trait, and the third also has sickle cell anaemia. Gemma is a bright girl who enjoys studying and is doing well at school. Both Gemma and her family, have an in-depth knowledge of her condition and competently manage it at home. Gemma has had several previous admissions to the ward in acute sickle cell crisis, and this is beginning to have an effect on both her social life and her schoolwork. She is starting to feel that her condition sets her apart from her friends, and while they are enjoying their teenage years, she always has to be careful of what she does to prevent either pain or anaemic crisis.

Following a recent chest infection, Gemma has again been admitted to the ward with an acute sickle cell crisis. She is obviously distressed, has acute shortness of breath and is in a great deal of pain. On examination it is noted that she is pyrexial at 38.4°C, tachycardic at 112 beats min⁻¹ and her respiratory rate = 32 breaths min⁻¹. Gemma complains of pain in both her feet and hands, which are obviously swollen. She also has acute abdominal pain and has been vomiting before admission. Owing to the pain she is having difficulty in finding a comfortable position in which to lie, and is becoming increasingly rude and aggressive, particularly to her parents whom she blames for her situation. The nursing staff are also receiving the brunt of her aggression.

Both Gemma's parents have accompanied her to the hospital, her brothers being looked after by a neighbour. They are upset that despite early treatment for her chest infection, they have failed to prevent a painful crisis, which has led to yet another admission to hospital. Gemma's aggression is also upsetting them as they state that she is usually 'sunny natured' and polite. They are also worried about the long-term prognosis for Gemma as she seems to be having an increasing number of painful crises.

Question one: Briefly describe the aetiology of sickle cell disease.

10 minutes

Question two: How would you manage Gemma's nursing care while she is on the ward?

20 minutes

Question three: Describe the possible complications that Gemma may experience as she enters adulthood.

10 minutes

Time Allocation: **40 minutes**

Answer to question one:
Briefly describe the aetiology of sickle cell disease.

Sickle cell disease is known as a haemaglobinopathy, in that the globin factor of the normal adult haemaglobin, HbA, is totally replaced by sickle haemaglobin, HbS (Campbell & McIntosh, 1998). Under conditions of decreased oxygen or dehydration, haemaglobin S changes its molecular structure and becomes distorted leading to 'sickling' of the red blood cells (Davies & Billson, 1996). The name derives from the subsequent crescent or 'sickle' shape of the cells.

The abnormal sickle shape of the cells means that they tend to stick or clump together more easily, which can lead to the changes outlined below.

The clinical manifestations of the disease are brought about by (Campbell & Glasper, 1995):

- Slowing of the blood due to increased viscosity and damage to the cells
- Capillary stasis
- Capillary obstruction and thrombosis

Client profiles in nursing: child health

Answer to question two:
How would you manage Gemma's nursing care while she is on the ward?

In the acute stages Gemma's nursing management is aimed at controlling the pain, treating the underlying infection, rehydration, adequate oxygenation and management of pyrexia. She may also require a blood transfusion if anaemic.

On admission, Gemma should have a quick but thorough assessment including baseline observations of TPR and BP. This will allow treatment to be prioritised and commenced as quickly as possible.

Following an assessment of Gemma's pain (see Profile 23, Melanie Court), analgesics such as pethidine or morphine should be administered, continuous infusion often being the preferred method (Campbell & Glasper, 1995; Anionwu, 1996). Careful positioning, in a position that Gemma finds comfortable, may also help to reduce the pain from swelling in the limbs. Early assessment and treatment of pain is important, to reduce Gemma's distress and aggression.

Treatment of the underlying cause of the crisis should be initiated immediately. In this case, IV antibiotics (see Profile 26, Stephanie Coles) should be administered to treat Gemma's chest infection. The hospital policy about the administration of IV medications should be followed when undertaking this procedure. Strict aseptic techniques should be adhered to as any further infection could lead to the crisis becoming more acute and possibly to death.

As Gemma has been vomiting, she may be dehydrated, which could lead to increased 'sickling' of the cells. Aspects of rehydration therapy should include administration of anti-emetics to control vomiting, and IV fluids. Haemodilution helps to control the sickling by diluting the viscous blood so Gemma should be encouraged to drink regularly once the vomiting is under control (Moules & Ramsey, 1998). An accurate record of fluid balance should be maintained.

To ensure adequate oxygenation, oxygen may be administered in the short-term. Gemma should remain on bed rest, which will reduce her oxygen require-ments and also reduce fatigue (Campbell & Glasper, 1995). Pulse oximetry should be carried out to assess oxygen saturation levels, while oxygen therapy is being provided (Day, 1998). Sitting Gemma up in bed, well supported by pillows, will allow for greater lung expansion and will assist her breathing.

On admission, it was noted that Gemma was pyrexial, so cooling measures should be commenced. These include nursing Gemma with the minimum of clothing and bedclothes, keeping the area cool and administering oral paracetamol. Her temperature should then be monitored and recorded at regular intervals.

If indicated by anaemia or uncontrolled hypoxia, Gemma might require a blood transfusion. The nurse will then be responsible for the management of the transfusion and recognition of any signs of complications or incompatibility (Smeltzer & Bare, 1992; Wong *et al.*, 1999):

- Before commencement of the infusion, baseline observations of temperature, pulse, respirations and BP will allow for comparison of vital signs while the blood is being transfused

- Blood group and type on the blood bag should be checked with the patient's records, as should the patient's name
- Once the transfusion is in progress, vital signs should be monitored at regular intervals, which allows for early detection of any signs of haemolytic reaction. These include chills, fever, low back pain, hypotension, headache and nausea
- Should any of these reactions occur the transfusion should be stopped immediately and the paediatrician notified

All aspects of care should be discussed with Gemma and her parents. Gemma may be unwilling to cooperate initially due to tiredness and irritability and the nursing staff should be aware of this and make allowances. Gemma and her parents should be encouraged to discuss the long-term prognosis, once the acute stage is over.

Answer to question three:
Describe the possible complications that Gemma may experience as she enters adulthood.

As Gemma moves into adulthood she may continue to have episodes of painful or anaemic crises. In the past she might not have survived to adulthood, but due to early detection of the disease, increased access to medical care, and education of children and parents more children are surviving longer. However, patients admitted frequently in crises continue to be at higher risk of early death (Anionwu, 1996). Complications in adulthood include, respiratory disease, progressive lung damage, cardiac disease, genitourinary abnormalities, hepatobiliary disease and neurological complications such as a stroke. Depending on the frequency of the crises, Gemma may also find that sickle cell has an impact on her psychosocial well-being (Woods, 1994). The incidence rate of depression has also been identified as being higher in children with sickle cell disease than that of their siblings (Lee *et al.*, 1996).

References

Anionwu, E. N. (1996). Sickle cell and thallassaemia: some priorities for nursing research. *Journal of Advanced Nursing*, 23, 583–586.

Campbell, A. G. M., & McIntosh, N. (1998). *Forfar and Arneil's Textbook of Paediatrics*, 5th edn. Harlow: Churchill-Livingstone.

Campbell, S., & Glasper, E. A. (1995). *Whaley and Wong's Children's Nursing*. London: Mosby.

Davies, A. E. M., & Billson, A. L. (1996). *Key Topics in Paediatrics*. Oxford: BIOS.

Day, J. (1998). Crisis management. *Nursing Times*, 94, 28–29.

Lee, E. J., Phoenix, D., Brown, W., & Jackson, B. S. (1997). A comparison study of children with sickle cell disease and their non-diseased siblings on hopelessness, depression, and perceived competence. *Journal of Advanced Nursing*, 25, 79–86.

Moules, T., & Ramsey, J. (1998). *The Textbook of Children's Nursing*. Cheltenham: Stanley Thornes.

Smeltzer, S. C., & Bare, B. C. (1992). *Brunner and Sudarth's Textbook of Medical Surgical Nursing*, 7th edn. Philadelphia: J. B. Lippincott.

Wong, D. L., Hockenberry-Eaton, M., Wilson, D., Winkelstein, M. L., Ahmann, E., & DiVito-Thomas, P.A. (1999). *Whaley & Wong's Nursing Care of Infants and Children*, 6th edn. St Louis: Mosby.

Woods, K. (1994, accessed: 27 July 2000). Sickle cell disease: beyond the pain a comprehensive approach to care. In Topics in primary care [http://uhs.bsd.uchicago.edu/uhs/topics/sickle.cell.html].

Further reading

See Profile 10 (Selina Robiero).

Meningococcal septicaemia and fluid balance

Debbi Atkinson

Caroline Davies, aged 14 years, had been experiencing 'flu-like' symptoms since attending the school disco last night. Since waking this morning, she had been feeling increasingly lethargic, hot and nauseated. As she got dressed, she noticed a rash had developed on her chest, abdomen and legs. She called her mother, who on discovering that the rash did not blanch to pressure called her GP. The GP arrived and after examining Caroline gave her cefotaxime IV. He explained that Caroline had meningococcal meningitis and called for an ambulance to take her and her parents to the nearest childrens' department.

On arrival at the childrens' ward, Caroline was weighed to calculate her drug dosages. Her weight was 50 kg and her vital signs were: heart rate = 115 beats min^{-1}, BP = 105/60 mmHg, temperature = 38.5°C, capillary refill time (CRT) = 4 s, respiratory rate = 32 breaths min^{-1} and partial saturation of arterial oxygen (SaO_2) = 88% in air. Caroline's rash had become more florid, but her skin was pale. She was prescribed 60% humidified oxygen via a facemask, which increased the SaO_2 to 94%.

Caroline's BP was now 75 mmHg systolic (a diastolic pressure cannot be heard), so 20 ml kg^{-1} of a colloid solution was administered IV, with little effect. CRT was now 6 s and Caroline was showing signs of central cyanosis. As a result, more colloid was prescribed totalling 80 ml kg^{-1}. This increased the BP to 90/50 mmHg. Emergency resuscitative equipment and drugs were brought to Caroline's bedside as her condition was unstable, and she might deteriorate further.

As Caroline's condition was worsening, the decision was made to transfer her to the paediatric intensive care unit for closer monitoring and more invasive treatment. The need for the transfer was explained to her and her parents, who have been with her since admission. They expressed their concerns for Caroline and for their other children. It was explained that close contacts are given prophylactic antibiotic cover and that this would be dispensed for them and Caroline's siblings.

Question one: With regard to Caroline's vital signs on admission, what are the normal parameters for a 14-year-old?

5 minutes

Question two: How is capillary refill time estimated and what is its significance?

10 minutes

Question three: How would one assess Caroline and use this information to plan and implement her care?

30 minutes

Time Allowance: **45 minutes**

Answer to question one:
With regard to Caroline's vital signs on admission, what are the normal parameters for a 14-year-old?

Box 25.1. Normal parameters.

Respiratory rate (> 12 years of age)	15–20 beats min^{-1}
Heart rate	60–100 beats min^{-1}
Systolic blood pressure	100–120 mmHg
Temperature	37°C
SaO$_2$	100% in air
CRT	< 2 s

(Mackaway-Jones *et al.*, 1997)

Answer to question two:
How is capillary refill time estimated and what is its significance?

- Lift the hand or foot (depending on the limb to be used) slightly above the level of the heart (so refill is not assisted by gravity)
- Apply blanching pressure on a digit for 5 s
- Release pressure; capillary refill (colour) should occur within 2 s

CRT indicates the state of blood flow to the periphery. A slower refill time (> 2 s) indicates poor skin perfusion as a consequence of capillary vasoconstriction. The capillaries vasoconstrict in an attempt to support failing blood pressure and is an early sign of shock. As vasoconstriction will occur when the peripheries are cold, the interpretations of CRT must be made in light of the ambient temperature (Mackaway-Jones et al., 1997).

Answer to question three:
How would you assess Caroline and use this information to plan and implement her care?

Assessment is best made following the ABC (airway, breathing, circulation) approach.

Initially the nurse should ascertain whether Caroline can maintain her own airway. If she is breathing spontaneously, then she should be sat in an upright position to aid chest expansion, and oxygen should be administered as prescribed via a facemask.

If Caroline's condition deteriorates, it may be necessary to intubate and ventilate her to give higher concentrations of oxygen than can be accurately administered via a facemask. If Caroline is intubated, then patency of the tube must be ensured by the application of suction (Dean, 1997). This prevents secretions obstructing the lumen of the tube. Careful fixation of the tube and support of the ventilator tubing is required so that the endotracheal tube (ETT) is not displaced.

The second aspect of respiratory assessment is to gauge whether Caroline is breathing adequately. If breathing is spontaneous, assess the rate, depth and pattern of breathing. Quick recognition of respiratory distress can avert a further rapid deterioration. If Caroline is ventilated, then observation of equal chest movement and auscultation of air entry to apices and bases helps confirm the correct position of the ETT. Chest radiography can also confirm that mechanical ventilation is taking place. Regular monitoring of the ventilator settings for airway pressure and oxygen requirements can help in detecting changes in lung function.

Neurological observations will need to be performed regularly on Caroline to assess the level of consciousness. For a detailed explanation of these observations, see Profile 9 (Jason King).

The initial assessment of Caroline's circulation is performed visually. This involves an assessment for oedema and colour. Oedema might indicate capillary leakage of plasma from the blood vessels into the tissues, which is an early event in shock (Nadel *et al.*, 1995). Colour changes could include pallor indicating peripheral constriction and/or cyanosis as a result of tissue hypoxia, which is a late event in shock (Nadel *et al.*, 1995). Caroline's CRT = 6 s. She is centrally cyanosed and is hypotensive despite receiving colloids, all of which combine to give a diagnosis of shock. The immediate treatment required is IV fluid replacement to increase the circulating volume and to perfuse peripheral tissues (Holland *et al.*, 1993; Nadel *et al.*, 1995).

Caring for Caroline's IV infusion involves assessing the patency of the IV access and observing for complications (as identified in Box 25.2, at least twice daily (Sadik & Elliott, 1999).

> **Box 25.2.** Potential complications of cannulation and intravenous therapy (adapted from Sadik & Elliott, 1999)
>
> - Infection: increased temperature, raised pulse, pus at site
> - Local inflammation: redness, swelling, tenderness, hardening of the vein
> - Extravasation: swelling, tenderness, oedema
> - Thrombophlebitis: see Local inflammation
> - Air embolism: sudden hypotension, tachycardia, cyanosis and decreased consciousness
> - Overhydration: dyspnoea, cough, confusion, decreased consciousness, generalised oedema

The nurse must calculate the fluid requirements to prevent hydration or circulatory overload (Table 28.1).

Table 28.1 Fluid requirements (Insley, 1996).

Body weight (kg)	Fluid (ml kg^{-1} day^{-1})
≤ 10	100–120
10–30	60–90
≥ 30	40–90

As Caroline weighs 50 kg, she requires between 40 and 90 ml kg^{-1} day^{-1}. This works out at:

$40 \times 50 = 2000$ ml
$90 \times 50 = 4500$ ml.

Caroline's fluid requirement per day is, therefore, between 2000 and 4500 ml.

A serious complication of Caroline's condition is disseminated intravascular coagulation (DIC). DIC occurs as a result of endotoxin release from pathogenic microorganisms, especially Gram-negative bacteria. DIC may result in depletion of platelets and clotting factors, leading to widespread haemorrhage and the deposition of fibrin clots in blood vessels of all sizes.

Subsequently clots in large arteries cause diverse ischaemia of major organs with subsequent death. The main sign is a petechial or purpuric rash and as this is a presenting sign of meningitis this might lead to confusion and a delay in diagnosis. Treatment is the administration of fresh frozen plasma and platelets, aiming at maintaining her fibrinogen level at 100–150 mg dl^{-1}. Heparin 500 units h^{-1} might need to be administered if thrombotic complications are present (Schlishtimann & Graber, 1999). The role of the nurse is to be aware of the possibility of DIC in the acutely ill child, to recognise indicative signs and to initiate immediate treatment. The consequences of DIC in children can vary enormously and are related to the vessels affected and the impact of subsequent ischaemia. In its most extreme form thrombosis of central and peripheral vessels can lead to gangrene, tissue necrosis and potential amputation of digits or limbs. However, this only happens in the minority of cases (Cahill-Aslip & McDermott, 1996).

Although the complications of meningitis are devastating, a recent innovation in the prevention of meningitis is the production of a drug called Neuprex, manufactured by Xoma in the USA. It has been noted to reduce the number of deaths from meningitis by up to 70% and may soon be on general prescription in the UK (Halle, 2000).

References

Cahill-Aslip, C., & McDermott, B. (1996). Hematologic critical care problems. In M. A. Q. Curley, J. B. Smith, & A. Moloney-Harman (eds), *Critical Care Nursing of Infants and Children* (793–818). London: W. B. Saunders.

Dean, B. (1997). Evidence-based suction management in Accident and Emergency: a vital component of airway care. *Accident and Emergency Nursing*, 5, 92–98.

Halle, M. (2000). Could this drug beat meningitis? *Daily Mail*, 4 April, 13.

Holland, J. A., Bryan, S., & Huff-Slankard, J. (1993). Nursing care of a child with meningococcemia. *Journal of Pediatric Nursing: Nursing Care of Children and Families*, 8, 211–216.

Insley, J (ed.) (1996). *A Paediatric Vade-Mecum*. London: Edward Arnold.

Mackaway-Jones, K., Molyneux, E., Phillips, B., & Wieteska, S. (eds) (1997). *Advanced Paediatric Life Support: The Practical Approach*. London: BMJ Publ.

Nadel, S., Habibi, P., & Levin, M. (1995). Management of meningococcal septicaemia. *Care of the Critically Ill*, 11, 33–38.

Sadik, R., & Elliott, D. E. (1999). Respiration and circulation. In R. Hogston, & P. M. Simpson (eds), *Foundations of Nursing Practice* (167–215). Basingstoke: Macmillan.

Schlishtimann, J., & Graber, M. (1999). *University of Ohio Family Practice Handbook*, 3rd edn.

Further reading

Association of the British Pharmaceutical Industry (1998). *Compendium of Data Sheets*. London: Datapharm.

Blumer, J. L. (ed.) (1998). *A Practical Guide to Pediatric Intensive Care*. London: Mosby.

Bradford, A. (1994). *Meningococcal meningitis. Intensive and Critical Care Nursing*, 10, 199–208.

Waterston, T., Platt, M. W., & Helms, P. (1997). *Paediatrics: Understanding Child Health*. Oxford: Oxford University Press.

Burns

Gill Campbell and Ruth Sadik

Stephanie Coles, is a 14-year-old who is expected to arrive at the Accident and Emergency department within the next 5 minutes. Along with her parents and two younger brothers, Stephanie has been involved in a house fire that occurred an hour ago while the family was asleep. The ambulance crew radio to the hospital that Stephanie is semiconscious but breathing spontaneously requiring 5 litres min^{-1} oxygen (O_2) to maintain saturation levels (SaO_2, i.e. the partial saturation of arterial oxygen) of 92%.

She has sustained partial and full-thickness burns to her right arm. There is some blistering of the skin across her chest and neck, and she has soot deposits around the nose and mouth. Stephanie was in a lot of pain and has been given a dose of morphine by the paramedic, based on an estimated body weight of 46 kg. An IV infusion of a colloid solution has been commenced, but, despite a rapid infusion, Stephanie's BP is deteriorating.

When Stephanie arrives in the department, her BP = 85/50 mmHg, pulse = 130 beats min^{-1}, respiration rate = 32 min^{-1}, SaO_2 = 88%. A second infusion of a colloid solution is commenced and her O_2 therapy increased to 10 l min^{-1}.

The circulation to her right hand appears impaired due to the tightening of a circumferential burn. An escharotomy is performed following which the circulation to the affected hand, although weak, is found to be returning.

An anaesthetist is called in view of the deposits around Stephanie's nose and mouth and her reduced level of consciousness. There are indications of smoke inhalation and she is electively intubated as ensuing oedema will make emergency intubation difficult if left.

Question one: What specific nursing assessments relating to her burns will Stephanie require?

45 minutes

Question two: Discuss the nurse's role before, during and following the administration of IV fluids and drugs.

20 minutes

Time Allocation: **1 hour 5 minutes**

Answer to question one:
What specific nursing assessments relating to her burns will Stephanie require?

Stephanie's airway is at risk as she has blistering to her neck and soot deposits around her nostrils, which are indicative of smoke inhalation. Smoke is itself an irritant with toxic hydrocarbons, carbon monoxide and cyanide. Stephanie requires immediate treatment with humidified oxygen and she should be observed for a dry cough and/or hoarseness. The nurse should expect Stephanie's sputum to contain black carbon specks.

If the inhalation is severe, as diagnosed by Stephanie's blood gases, she may require bronchial lavage and/or treatment for poisoning by carbon monoxide or cyanide. Close observation of Stephanie's respiratory rate, effort, depth and rhythm will be required.

Immediately following a burn, there is an increased dilation and permeability of capillaries and a shift of fluid from the vascular compartment to the interstitial space, causing oedema and a reduced intravascular volume (Coleshaw *et al.*, 1997).

To detect hypovolaemic shock quickly, the nurse needs to observe the factors given in Table 26.1.

Table 26.1. Indicators of hypovolaemic shock.

Nursing observations	Indications of hypovolaemic shock
Pulse	tachycardia
Blood pressure	hypotension
Capillary refill time (CRT)	> 2 s
Temperature	peripheral hypothermia
Urinary output	< 1 ml kg^{-1} h^{-1}

The nurse needs to record pulse, BP, capillary refill time and temperature every 15–30 min (Kelly, 1994). Neurovascular observation of Stephanie's arm must also be performed to prevent compartment syndrome (see Profile 17, Sian Williams).

The administration of an IV colloid fluid is vital, and an accurate fluid balance must be maintained. However, the fluid requirements for a burnt child are calculated using a different formula to that found in Profile 25 (Caroline Davis). The position and percentage of skin burnt, along with an assessment of severity, must be performed to use one of the various formulae currently used, an example of which is in Box 26.1.

Box 26.1. Fluid calculation for children with > 10% of their skin burnt (Insley, 1996).

- Colloid solution equal to the normal plasma volume for every 15% of burnt skin
- Half to be given in 8 h and the remainder over the rest of the 24-h period
- Rate may need to be adjusted to maintain a urine output of 1 ml kg^{-1} h^{-1}
- Oral fluids should be reduced by 25%

The calculation is made from the time that Stephanie was burnt rather than the admission time. Whichever formula is used to assess Stephanie's fluid requirements, fresh plasma or a colloid substitute will be the infusion of choice.

The percentage of skin burnt is calculated as shown in Table 26.2.

Table 26.2. Calculation of skin percentages burnt.

The following areas are the same percentage for all children:
  Front of neck: 1
  Back of neck: 1
  Front of each upper arm: 2
  Back of each upper arm: 2
  Front of each lower arm: 1.5
  Back of each lower arm: 1.5
  Back or front of each hand: 1.5
  Front of chest: 13
  Back: 13
  Front of abdomen: 2.5
  Genitalia: 1
  Each buttock: 2.5
  Upper or lower surface of each foot: 1.75

The following areas change with age (Beattie et al., 1997)

	Age (years)				
	0	1	5	10	15
0.5 of the head	9.50	8.50	6.50	5.50	4.50
0.5 of one thigh	2.75	3.25	4.00	4.50	4.75
0.5 of one leg	2.50	2.50	2.75	3.0	3.25

Box 26.2. Definition of burn thickness (Campbell & Glasper, 1995; Beattie et al., 1997).

- Superficial burns: of minor significance, characterised by erythema only. Heal quickly and do not usually result in a scar. Can be very painful
- Superficial partial-thickness burns: erythema plus blisters, some of which may burst. Pain and healing as for superficial burns
- Deep partial-thickness burns: the distinguishing feature here is that where the blisters burst the underlying tissue contains 'white' areas that indicate deep tissue involvement. The child's ability to feel in this area will be decreased and the wound is more prone to scarring
- Full-thickness burns: area burnt is completely white, leathery and has no sensation. Thrombosed veins might be present in the burn wound. Surgical intervention may be indicated. Once the burns have occurred, every system in the body may become involved. While superficial nerve endings are destroyed, they are hypersensitive on the wound edges. Decreased blood supply and the inflammatory process may, conversely, lead to deep pain within the burnt area

---

Water, plasma proteins and electrolytes (principally sodium and potassium) are lost through the burn and fluid requirement is, therefore, increased. Fluid losses are further complicated by increased capillary permeability and subsequent oedema in unaffected sites such as the gastrointestinal tract and brain. The aim of this treatment is to maintain a urine output of 1–2 ml kg^{-1} per h (Beattie *et al.*, 1997).

Pain will cause Stephanie a lot of distress as partial-thickness burns expose nerve endings at the skin surface (Coleshaw *et al.*, 1997) (see Box 26.2 for a definition of partial-thickness burns). As she may have been in shock at the time of the injury, diminished blood supply to the muscles would mean that initial analgesics should have been administered via the IV route (ALSG, 1997). In cases where the initial route is unknown, the nurse should be cautious in subsequent administration; as the child's perfusion improves, opiates that have been administered intramuscularly may be absorbed. Analgesic support might be continued successfully with the older child by the use of entonox (Kelly, 1994), and this would be especially useful during dressing changes.

Concise assessment of Stephanie's pain plus accurate evaluation of the analgesic's effectiveness not only will make her pain free, but also will reduce her anxiety (for pain assessment, see Profile 23, Melanie Court).

Once burns damage the integrity of the skin, it no longer acts as a barrier to infection, thermoregulation is altered and fluid is lost (Coleshaw *et al.*, 1997). An accurate assessment of Stephanie's burn will need to be made as a baseline, so that future healing or tissue breakdown can be gauged.

All dressing changes will need to be carried out aseptically and with effective analgesic cover. The type of dressings and treatments should be under the guidance of a specialist burns team. To prevent infection, prophylactic antibiotics will be commenced. It is the nurse's responsibility to check whether Stephanie is allergic to these drugs and to administer them in accordance with national and hospital policies.

Body heat can be lost due to impairment of thermoregulatory function and to increased evaporation of fluid from the burn surface (Coleshaw *et al.*, 1997). Accurate monitoring of Stephanie's core and peripheral temperatures is required to assess the extent of vasoconstriction. The ambient temperature of Stephanie's room needs to be kept at 30°C following her injury to prevent hypothermia (Coleshaw *et al.*, 1997).

As stated above, in full-thickness burns all body systems become involved as summarised in Box 26.3.

Box 26.3. Effect of burns on body systems.

- Cardiovascular system:
  - anaemia: red cell destruction by heat, loss of red blood cells through damaged capillaries, direct bleeding from the wound both initially and during treatments, and potential bone marrow depression accompanying infection
  - burn shock: involves a 50% decrease in cardiac output as a result of large fluid losses through the burn process. In the majority of cases, children can compensate for this and cardiac output returns to normal spontaneously within 36 h
- Respiratory system: increased pulmonary tissue permeability and the effects of smoke inhalation may lead to pulmonary oedema
- Gastrointestinal system: children are more prone than adults to develop duodenal ulceration, known as Curling's ulcers, 3–4 weeks post-burn (Wong et al., 1999). As a result, severely burnt children may be given cimetidine IV as prophylaxis. Paralytic ileus might also develop within the first 3 post-burn days and as such may require the passage of a nasogastric tube (see Profile 23, Melanie Court). Glycogen breakdown occurs as part of the stress reaction to severe burns and within the first 24 h the body stores may be fully depleted. Protein breakdown is also accelerated and this requires an increase of 1.5 times the normal calorie requirement (Stephanie's normal requirement is 2200 calories day^{-1}) and two-to-three times the normal protein requirement (Stephanie's normal requirement is 46 g day^{-1}) (Insley, 1996). This may need to be delivered parenterally if oral fluids are not tolerated (see Profile 6, Nathan Simms)
- Renal: as a result of fluid movement from the blood vessels to the tissues, vasoconstriction occurs leading to reduced renal plasma flow and decreased glomerular filtration. Blood urea and creatinine levels increase as a result of tissue breakdown and oliguria. Haematuria might also be evident as a result of red cell haemolysis and renal failure may ensue if fluid replacement is ineffective
- Central nervous system: cerebral oedema may result in hallucinations, personality change and possible fitting. The effects of cerebral oedema are exacerbated by hypoxaemia, electrolyte imbalance and the adverse effects of various drugs

Answer to question 2:
Discuss the nurse's role before, during and following the administration of IV drugs and fluids.

Before:

- Ensure that the nurse's knowledge of universal precautions is current
- Check the prescription chart for the correct:
  - child's name
  - drug or fluid
  - dosage or amount
  - route
  - date and time
  - duration of administration
  - expiry date
  - ensure fluids are particle free
- Ensure that the nurse understands the action of the drug, the correct dosage and the possible side-effects (a child-appropriate pharmacological text should be used if there is any doubt (e.g. RCPCH, 1999)
- IV drugs and fluids should be checked by two nurses
- Correct preparation of the drug including consideration of the displacement volume
- Identify the child using an identification tag or a competent adult (e.g. parent) if no tag is in place
- Ascertain known allergies
- Check cannula patency (see Profile 25, Caroline Davis)

During:

- Assess the child throughout the procedure for:
  - pain and discomfort
  - possible anaphylaxis including:
    - erythema
    - tachycardia
    - rhinitis, itching or sneezing
    - hypotension
    - dysrhythmia
    - laryngeal oedema
    - bronchospasm
    - nausea or vomiting
    - diarrhoea
    - headache
    - seizures

Following:

- Sign the prescription chart that the drug has been given or that the fluid has been commenced
- Dispose of sharps appropriately
- Check the child's condition 20 min later to confirm that there are no adverse reactions

References

Advanced Life Support Group (1997). *Advanced Paediatric Life Support*, 2nd edn. London: BMJ Publ.

Beattie, T. F., Hendry, G. M., & Duguid, K. P. (1997). *Pediatric Emergencies*. London: Mosby-Wolfe.

Campbell, S., & Glasper, E. A. (eds) (1995). *Whaley and Wong's Children's Nursing*. London: Mosby.

Coleshaw, S., Reilly, S., & Irving, N. (1997). Management of burns. *Paediatric Nursing*, 9, 29–36.

Insley, J. (ed.) (1996). *A Paediatric Vade-Mecum*, 13th edn. London: Edward Arnold.

Kelly, H. (1994). Initial nursing assessment and management of burn-injured children. *British Journal of Nursing*, 3, 54–59.

Royal College of Paediatrics and Child Health (1999). *Medicines for Children*. London: RCPCH.

Wong, D. L., Hockenberry-Eaton, M., Wilson, D., Winkelstein, M. L., Ahmann, E., & DiVito-Thomas, P. A. (1999). *Whaley & Wong's Nursing Care of Infants and Children*, 6th edn. St Louis: Mosby.

Further reading

Graber, M. A. (n.d., accessed 24 July 2000). Emergency medicine: burns, cold, and thermal injury [http://www.vh.org/Providers/ClinRef/FPHandbook/Chapter01/23-1.htm].

Continuous ambulatory peritoneal dialysis

Debbie Atkinson

Joseph Feinnes is a 15-year-old only child who lives with his parents. When he was 10 years old, he was diagnosed as having chronic pyelonephritis, leading to end-stage renal failure. This has been treated with continuous ambulatory peritoneal dialysis (CAPD). Initially Joseph's parents worked with him in performing his CAPD, but in the past 18 months he has managed his CAPD independently.

Joseph is admitted to the adolescent unit following a 1-week history of low-grade pyrexia, lethargy and clouding of his dialysate fluid, accompanied by abdominal tenderness, especially during inflow of dialysate fluid.

On admission, Joseph is reluctant to discuss his dialysis and refuses to perform his own CAPD while on the ward.

According to his parents, Joseph is usually a happy, sociable boy, but now he appears quiet and withdrawn, and he does not wish to attend the games room or watch television, preferring to stay in his side room alone.

The plan of nursing care arranged for Joseph incorporates administering antibiotic therapy and re-evaluating his CAPD procedure.

Question one: Explain the difference between osmosis and diffusion.
10 minutes

Question two: Identify what peritoneal dialysis is.
10 minutes

Question three: Briefly describe the nursing care you would give Joseph while on your ward.
15 minutes

Question four: What strategies could you use to encourage Joseph to become involved in his care?
15 minutes

Time Allocation: **50 minutes**

Answer to question one:
Explain the difference between osmosis and diffusion.

Osmosis is the passive movement of **water** across a semipermeable membrane from a solution of lower concentration of particles to a solution of higher concentration. Whereas diffusion is the random movement of **particles** from an area of greater concentration to an area of lower concentration. When diffusion occurs across a semipermeable membrane, the particles that move are dependent on the size of the pores within the membrane (i.e. large particles such as proteins or glucose are generally too large to pass unaided through a membrane) (Tortora & Grabowski, 2000).

Answer to question two:
Identify what peritoneal dialysis is.

In health, the kidneys are responsible for filtration, selective re-absorption and secretion of solutes. This mechanism enables the pH of the blood and body fluids to remain within normal parameters.

Peritoneal dialysis is used when the kidneys are no longer able to function. This leads to the signs, symptoms and reasons given in Box 27.1 (adapted from Tortora & Grabowski, 2000).

Box 27.1. Signs, symptoms and reasons.

- Oedema: failure to excrete sodium and water
- Acidosis: failure to excrete hydrogen ions
- Increased levels of non-protein nitrogen substances, especially urea: failure to excrete metabolic waste products
- Increased potassium levels: failure to excrete potassium
- Anaemia: lack of renal erythropoietic factor
- Osteomalacia: kidneys cannot convert vitamin D to 1,25-dihydrooxy-calciferol (its active form) to allow for calcium absorption

---

The procedure of peritoneal dialysis is reliant on osmosis and diffusion of water and solutes across the peritoneum, which acts as a semipermeable membrane.

The dialysate fluid will contain high concentrations of solutes that need to be absorbed and low concentrations of solutes which need to be excreted from the body. For example, the dialysate fluid may contain glucose to allow for movement of water, or low potassium levels to allow for excretion of excess potassium.

A permanent silastic catheter is inserted via the abdominal wall into the peritoneal cavity. Once healing has occurred, sterile dialysate fluid is allowed to flow into the cavity where it remains for some time before being drained out. The time that fluid remains in the peritoneal cavity will depend on the reason for dialysis and may vary from 30 min to 5 h (Moules and Ramsay, 1998) before being drained off and the cycle repeated. The two main methods of implementing PD are:

- CAPD: allows for continuous dialysis while Joseph continues his normal daily activities. The dwell times are usually 4–6 h allowing four or five exchanges a day. After the solution has been instilled, the bag is clamped off and placed in a compartment in the child's clothing, or strapped to the abdomen. Drainage can be performed during a normal school break time by everting the bag, unclamping it and allowing gravity to assist. Dwell time can be shortened throughout the day to fit in with normal activity and then increased overnight (Moules and Ramsay, 1998)
- Continuous cycling peritoneal dialysis (CCPD): machine used to deliver the exchanges automatically at night

The potential complications of PD are:

- Catheter obstruction: ensure tubing is free from kinks
- Catheter site leakage: weigh dressings to estimate amount. Notify the doctor
- Infection: peritonitis is common and can be prevented by strict hygiene measures at all times. Observe dialysate for signs of infection. Report any incidences of abdominal pain and fever
- Breathing difficulty due to the abdomen splinting the diaphragm: encourage deep breathing, elevate the bed head
- Fluid and electrolyte balance: monitor input and output

Answer to question three:
Briefly describe the nursing care you would give Joseph while on your ward.

Despite being admitted with a possible diagnosis of peritonitis, Joseph will continue to require his CAPD. To ensure that his infection does not progress further, it is the nurse's responsibility to ensure that all procedures involving Joseph's CAPD catheter are carried out aseptically. While undertaking Joseph's dialysis, the nurse has the opportunity to informally re-educate Joseph about his own technique, stressing the importance of hand washing and non-touch technique.

Antibiotics have been prescribed for Joseph that will involve them being administered IV or intra-peritoneally. Before these are given it is the nurse's responsibility to check that Joseph is not allergic to these drugs and that they are given in accordance with the hospital policy.

Pain from the abdominal infection might cause Joseph distress. Adequate, frequent analgesics must be given and their effectiveness assessed. Although there are several tools that could be used to assess adolescent pain, one example would be the PATCh (Pain Assessment Tool for Children) tool devised by Quershi & Buckingham (1994). This incorporates a numeric scale, descriptors of pain and behaviour, a body outline, and a face scale.

Owing to the inflammatory process involved in peritonitis, the increased permeability of the peritoneum will result in a rapid decrease in Joseph's plasma protein levels (leading to poor healing). It is important that dietary advice is sought as he requires a high protein diet and may not feel like eating. Joseph should be consulted about what food he likes and dislikes and about meal timings. By involving Joseph and his family in such issues, not only is it increasing their knowledge of his dietary requirements, but also it increases the likelihood of his compliance (Canam, 1993).

Constipation is to be avoided as an impacted bowel can cause the catheter to migrate upwards in the peritoneum. Ideally, Joseph's diet will avoid this, but if constipation does occur then the use of an aperient such as lactulose should be considered.

Answer to question four:
What strategies could you use to encourage Joseph to become involved in his care?

Attempt to engage Joseph in a discussion about how he feels. This could be on a one-to-one basis. Stressing that this conversation is strictly confidential may encourage Joseph to discuss issues or problems he may not wish others to know. A discussion of this nature should be conducted in a quiet place with no time limits or distractions. Peers are very important to adolescents (Farelly, 1994) and Joseph should be reassured that his friends can visit him and that a close link with his school will be maintained so that he does not become disadvantaged in preparatory work for examinations.

Joseph's reluctance to participate in his care may be due to anxiety, which could be attributed to hospitalisation restricting his autonomy, or embarrassment in case he is performing his CAPD incorrectly. Reassurance and re-education about his CAPD procedure should be given in a supportive manner. Allowing Joseph to plan his day and who visits him, as well as personalising his bed space, might help him reassert his autonomy and gain 'decisional' control whereby he makes the sort of decisions he is used to making for himself (Ellis, 1996).

References

Canam, C. (1993). Common adaptive tasks facing parents of children with chronic conditions. *Journal of Advanced Nursing*, 18, 46–53.

Ellis, P. A. (1996). Altered body image in patients on CAPD. *Professional Nurse*, 11, 537–538.

Farelly, R. (1994). The special care needs of the adolescent in hospital. *Nursing Times*, 90, 31–33.

Moules, T., & Ramsay, J. (1998). *The Textbook of Children's Nursing*. Cheltenham: Stanley Thornes.

Quershi, J., & Buckingham, S. (1994). A pain assessment tool for all children. *Paediatric Nursing*, 6, 11–13.

Tortora, J., & Grabowski, S. R. (2000). *Principles of Anatomy and Physiology*. New York: Wiley.

Further reading

Wong, D. L., Hockenberry-Eaton, M., Wilson, D., Winkelstein, M. L., Ahmann, E., & DiVito-Thomas, P. A. (1999). *Whaley and Wong's Nursing Care of Infants and Children*, 6th edn. St Louis: Mosby.

Adolescent with anorexia nervosa

Leigh F. Caws and Ruth Sadik

Elisa Cromwell is a 15-year-old monozygotic twin giving great cause for concern to her family because of her state of health and mental well being. Her mother is concerned about Elisa's lack of menstrual periods and her apparent weight loss, and when she persuaded her to be weighed on the bathroom scales at home she was shocked to find that she had lost 10 kg, her weight falling to 44 kg during the past 3 months.

Elisa's twin sister, Ellen, weighs in at 56 kg and is 165 cm in height. The girls live with their mother and their brother, Tim, who is 13 years old, in a four-bedroomed detached house in the suburbs of the city. Their father recently left the family home to live with another woman after he and his wife became increasingly estranged, and the couple has commenced divorce proceedings. The children still see their father at least twice a week and continue to have good relationships with both parents.

Elisa is a high achiever at school and hopes to get good grades for her GCSEs. She is a popular member of her class, but has become more reluctant to socialise with her friends outside school. Instead, she appears to spend most evenings in her room studying or watching television and her relationship with her sister has become more strained.

At mealtimes, there is often confrontation with her mother over Elisa's reluctance to eat, and if her father is present he tends to side with Elisa, apparently failing to acknowledge his wife's concerns.

Question one: Define anorexia nervosa, outlining current theories relating to its cause.

10 minutes

Question two: Describe the diagnostic features of anorexia nervosa.

10 minutes

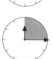

Question three: Rationalise Elisa's behaviour with what is known of anorexia nervosa.

15 minutes

Question four: Using a problem-solving approach, rationalise the nursing assessment one would make on Elisa and her family. Use current theories of anorexia nervosa that recognise the complicated interplay between social, psychological and physiological factors associated with growing up.

30 minutes

Time Allowance: **1 hour 5 minutes**

Answer to question one:
Define anorexia nervosa, outlining current theories relating to its cause.

Anorexia can be defined as a loss of appetite for psychological reasons (Halek, 1994). It is characterised by severe weight loss, over activity, decreased sleep and flattened emotion (Gelazis & Kempe, 1996). Frequently, it is confused with bulimia, where the individual concerned alternates periods of binge eating with purgation. While there are differences, there are also links with shared extreme concerns about shape and weight. These concerns or 'overvalued ideas' are, according to Lemme (1996), peculiar to people with eating disorders, and are associated with emotional, rather than rational belief.

Various theories have been put forward to explain the cause of this mental health phenomenon:

- Biological theories hypothesise that eating disturbances may originate from hypothalamic, hormonal, neurotransmitter, genetic or biochemical disorders (Halek, 1994)
- Psychodynamic/analytical, where the individual has never developed mature coping skills or regresses to pre-pubertal problem-coping skills to deal with difficulties, feelings such as anger, or the normal transition to adulthood. Gelazis and Kempe (1996: 670) noted that as anorexia frequently occurs at adolescence and may be accompanied with amenorrhoea, it might be associated with sexual problems or the repudiation of sexuality. This reluctance to gain independence may be related to child-rearing practices that ignore the child's demands in favour of the mother's desires. The developing child fails to discriminate its inner feelings (Howe et al., 1999), acquires a sense of self importance and cannot separate from parents and interact successfully with peers
- Cognitive theories revolve around the development of a distorted body image and irrational beliefs and thoughts. The adolescent believes that they are 'too fat', even when they are obviously emaciated. In contrast to the belief that people with anorexia do not like food, many spend hours pre-occupied with cooking and preparing meals for others (Casey, 1997)
- Socio-cultural theories propose that anorexia occurs more frequently in families where parents are controlling and impose high expectations on their children, with resultant conflict. In the West there is also an overemphasis on physical attractiveness being defined by thinness
- Behavioural theorists postulate that it may start with the decision to lose weight, which leads to the individual gaining satisfaction from the suppression of hunger. Fear of weight gain results in a preoccupation with remaining thin (Gelazis & Kempe, 1996)
- Family systems theory suggest that there are definable characteristics of the family containing an anorexic child (Johnson, 1997). The father is viewed as passive, the mother controlling and the child as over-dependent. Family interaction patterns involve enmeshment, overprotectiveness, rigidity and lack of conflict resolution

Treatment and interventions will depend on the personal theoretical beliefs of the team involved in Elisa's care, her needs and those of her family.

Answer to question two:
Describe the diagnostic features of anorexia nervosa.

Anorexia nervosa has been identified with a 'nervous loss of appetite'. However, young people like Elisa maintain a strong interest in food and, more importantly, they feel that their appetite is too powerful. They attempt to exert control over these powerful urges through constant vigilance and following the most stringent rules of when, and what, they may eat (Lemme, 1996). Conventional dieting with the reduction or omission of sweet, high-calorie carbohydrate foods often precedes the pursuit of thinness. Eventually, the individual becomes an expert in the calorie content of foods, but sets themselves unreasonably low daily caloric intakes (restrictive anorexia).

If Elisa found herself acquiescing to her mother's demands at mealtimes, she may fear losing control and 'falling to pieces'.

There are various diagnostic classifications for mental health problems and the ones most widely used in the UK are the Diagnostic Statistic Manual (DSM)-IV edn (Frances, 1994) and the International Classification of Diseases (ICD), 10th edn (WHO, 1992). They identify the defining criteria of anorexia nervosa as given in Box 28.1.

Box 28.1. Comparison of classification systems.	
DSM-IV (1994)	ICD-10 (1992)
Individual refuses to maintain a body weight over a minimum 'average expected body weight' (AEBW) calculated on the basis of age, gender and height	Body weight $\leq$ 15% of expected
Disturbance in the individual's perception of own weight, size or shape	Body image distortion and fear of fatness
Intense fear of gaining weight is experienced	Self-induced weight loss. Avoidance of fattening foods
Absence of three consecutive menstrual periods	Abnormalities of hypothalamic pituitary–gonadal axis, amenorrhoea, decreased libido, increased growth hormone. Delayed onset of puberty

These classification systems acknowledge the need to differentiate between individuals who refuse to eat and primary anorexia (Lemme, 1996). Primary anorexia can be further subdivided into 'restrictive anorexia' and 'bulimic anorexia'. In the former, the young person severely restricts their intake, while in the latter, strict dieting is alternated with vomiting (Lemme, 1996). Rigorous exercise and abuse of laxatives or diuretics also serve to regulate body weight (Steinhausen, 1994). Mood swings, irritability, insomnia and depression usually manifest as a result of starvation. Other physical signs of advanced anorexia nervosa (Box 28.2) include bradycardia, hypotension and hypothermia (Steinhausen, 1994), but these clinical manifestations can be masked by the effects of profound anaemia.

Box 28.2. Consequences of anorexia on body systems.

- Neurological: EEG abnormalities, seizures, peripheral neuritis
- Cardiovascular: bradycardia, ↓ BP, ↓ heart size, EEG abnormalities, oedema
- Metabolic: dehydration, hypoglycaemia, ↑ cholesterol, ↑ amylase, ↓ plasma proteins, ↓ potassium, ↓ calcium, ↓ magnesium
- Endocrine: ↑ growth hormone, ↓ gonadotrophins
- Haematologic: iron deficiency anaemia, hypocellular marrow
- Gastrointestinal: swollen salivary glands, dental caries, ↓gastric emptying, constipation
- Renal: partial diabetes insipidus, renal failure
- Musculoskeletal: osteoporosis, stress fractures, ↓growth, cramps
- Other: hypothermia, infections, lanugo, increased risk of abortion and decreased birth weight (if pregnant)

Answer to question three:
Rationalise Elisa's behaviour with what is known of anorexia nervosa.

Elisa is trapped in a body that she perceives as fat even though it is clearly emaciated. She is also trapped in thoughts that revolve obsessively around food, shape and weight, which are subsequently intimately linked to how she feels about herself.

Elisa originally weighed 54 kg (~50th centile) and lost 10 kg; her twin sister weighs 56 kg (~50th centile) and is 165 cm in height (~75th centile). One must assume that the sisters are of a similar height.

Elisa's current weight is 19% less than one would expect for a female of her age and height, and her periods have ceased. Therefore, she fulfils at least two of the guidelines of the classification of anorexia nervosa.

Eating disorders are more likely to manifest in adolescents because of the convergence of physical changes and psycho-social challenges with which the adolescent must cope (Steinhauser, 1994). Attie et al. (1990) suggested that the increase in body fat experienced by females at this developmental milestone can bring about dieting behaviour as the changes in physical appearance, bodily feelings and reproductive status require reorganisation and trans-formation of the body image. Elisa's condition may also be the result of being part of a dysfunctional family in the light of the recent parental separation and as Minuchin (1984) pointed out, the role of the anorectic daughter may serve to divert attention from impending family conflict, thus increasing her dependence on the family as a whole. The father appears to side with Elisa about her reluctance to eat, overriding the mother's concerns, which may serve as evidence of achieving her dependence on both parents. Elisa has become socially withdrawn, with probable mood swings, irritability and depression. She appears to have a distorted drive to achieve thinness, control of body shape and bodily functions not only through starvation, but also through excessive exercise, inducing vomiting and possibly by taking laxatives/diuretics.

Answer to question four:

Using a problem-solving approach, rationalise the nursing assessment one would make on Elisa and her family. Use current theories of anorexia nervosa that recognise the complicated interplay between social, psychological and physiological factors associated with growing up.

The assessment of Elisa will set the tone for the remainder of the interactions with her and her family. According to Buckley *et al.* (1995), it provides an opportunity to deal with parental fears and misunderstandings, supports their desire to be good parents and encourages them actively to participate in their daughter's care. Holyoake and Jenkins (1998) suggested that the nursing assessment should include information about the emotional, social, physiological and psychological domains of the client to implement 'Passive Activity Time' (PAT), a nursing intervention developed for young people with eating disorders. The framework for this model is outlined in Table 28.1.

Table 28.1. Assessment criteria for PAT (Holyoake & Jenkins, 1998).

Domains	Assessment criteria
Emotional	irrational fears in relation to self ability to form appropriate emotional responses to stress
Social	abnormal relationships: age-appropriate relationships with the same sex inappropriate relationships with opposite sex out-of-home activities
Physiological	how much weight lost? classification of malnutrition, e.g. is it sudden or long standing weight loss? physical history: posture, muscle, nervous control, hair, skin mouth, lips, gums teeth, eyes, sickness
Psychological	history of obsessional traits? early feeding difficulties? family beliefs about food beliefs about food/ power dynamics/relationships mood/feelings about self and others

Elisa's problems are identified and an assessment with rationales using the PAT model is described in Table 28.2.

Client profiles in nursing: child health

Table 28.2. Elisa's assessment criteria.

Domains	Problems	Assessment and rationale
Emotional	parental separation impending divorce father has a new partner school work and GCSEs	establish Elisa's feelings and fears to her parent's separation and how this will affect her what are her feelings towards her father's new partner? identify Elisa's academic goals and expectations so that she can be helped to succeed in achieving realistic goals. This in turn will give her self-confidence
Social	high personal academic goals	explore areas of interest to Elisa in order to plan care, which incorporates activities and interests that require minimal physical activity to conserve energy for growth and keep her mind occupied
	becoming socially withdrawn from peers and family decline of relationship with twin	discuss the nature of her friendships so that she can feel free to express concerns explore family relationships and attitudes towards one another in order to assess family dynamics and functions
Physiological	lost 10 kg in weight in 3 months	calculate Elisa's healthy weight and weigh once/twice weekly without informing Elisa of the results as this information may prove too over-whelming for her as 1 kg week^{-1} is the expected weight gain (Holyoake & Jenkins, 1998).
	breathless on climbing stairs and tachycardia. Vomiting on occasions	assess for skin pallor/cyanosis, pulse and rate/depth of breathing as anaemia may lead to heart failure assess precipitating factors (behavioural), frequency and nature of vomiting. As there is a risk of dehydration and electrolyte imbalance, assist in taking blood for urea and electrolytes observe the teeth, gums, tongue and lips for signs of acid erosion from vomiting
	pressure risk due to poor nutrition and imposed limited activity	observe skin at pressure sites for redness and breakdown due to poor nutritional status
Psychological	refusal to eat enough to maintain weight	find out what foods interest Elisa, as these may be a starting point to eating, and what foods she dislikes, to avoid presenting these to her discover her normal eating patterns and preferences as this can act as a baseline, then try to establish what her eating patterns were when she was well. This could act as a goal to work towards or conversely to modify eating patterns explore beliefs and values about food to establish Elisa's feelings about food
	early onset of depression	discuss her personal and family history to identify early feeding difficulties, obsessional traits and influences on eating to establish a reason for the illness

References

Attie, I., Brooks-Gunn, F., & Peterson, A. C. (1990). A developmental perspective on eating disorders and eating problems. In M. Lewis, & S. M. Miller (eds), *Handbook of Developmental Psychopathology* (409–420). New York: Plenum.

Buckley, P. F., Bird, J., & Harrison, G. (1995). *Examination Notes in Psychiatry*. London: Butterworth-Heinemann.

Casey, P. R. (1997). *A Guide to Psychiatry in Primary Care*. Petersfield: Wrightson Biomedical.

Frances, A. (ed.) (1994). *Diagnostic and Statistical Manual of Mental Disorders*, 4th edn. Washington, DC: American Psychiatric Association.

Gelazis, R. S., & Kempe, A. (1996). Therapy with clients with eating disorders. In C. K. Beck, R. P. Rawlins, & S. R. Williams (eds), *Mental Health: Psychiatric Nursing* (662–680). St Louis: Mosby.

Halek, C. (1994). Eating and appetite. In H. Wright, & M. Giddey (eds), *Mental Health Nursing: From First Principles to Professional Practice*. London: Chapman & Hall.

Holyoake, D. D., & Jenkins, M. (1998). PAT: advanced nursing interventions for eating disorders. *British Journal of Nursing*, 7, 596–600.

Howe, D., Brandon, M., Hinings, D., & Schofield, G. (1999). *Attachment Theory, Child Maltreatment and Family Support*. Basingstoke: Macmillan.

Johnson, B. S. (1997). *Adaptation and Growth: Psychiatric-Mental Health Nursing*. New York: Lippincott.

Lemme, A. (1996). *Introduction to Psychopathology*. London: Sage.

Minuchin, S. (1984). *Family Kaleidoscope*. Cambridge MA: Harvard University Press.

Steinhausen, H. C. (1994). Anorexia and bulimia nervosa. In M. Rutter, E. Taylor, & L. Hersov (eds), *Child and Adolescent Psychiatry* (425–428). Oxford: Blackwells.

World Health Organisation (1992). Tenth Revision of the international classification of diseases. Chapter V. (F): Mental and Behavioural Disorder. *Clinical Descriptions and Diagnostic Guidelines*. Geneva: WHO.

Further reading

Brumberg, J. (1988). *Fasting Girls*. Cambridge, MA: Harvard University Press.